How to Quiet Your Mind in a Loud World

AN EXPLORATION OF MISOPHONIA FOR ADULTS AND TEENS

Shaylynn Hayes-Raymond

Published by Misophonia International
Columbia, Missouri

Distributed by Imperceptions Press

Cover art and print/eBook design
by Imperceptions Press

Edited by Harrison Porter

Hardcover ISBN: 978-1-990467-41-7

Print ISBN: 978-1-990467-39-4

Ebook ISBN: 978-1-990467-40-0

A

misophonia

matters

PUBLICATION

TABLE OF CONTENTS

INTRODUCTION
WHO THIS BOOK IS FOR

How To Quiet Your Mind in a Loud World is the spiritual successor of Shaylynn Hayes-Raymond's 2015 book *Full of Sound and Fury*. This book is especially geared toward adults and teens with misophonia, and provides an over-view of the condition, the culture surrounding it, as well as practical coping skills. For those who have already read *Misophonia Matters* and *Full of Sound and Fury*, this book may seem repetitive, so it is recommended for new readers interested in the condition. *How To Quiet Your Mind in a Loud World* is an honest examination of misophonia by a clinician who has the disorder herself.

This book is written with adults and teenagers with misophonia in mind. Parents and clinicians may be interested in instead reading *Misophonia Matters*, which is a more in-depth plan for coping with misophonia that takes less of a narrative approach to the disorder. However, there is nothing wrong with choosing this book if that is what you prefer. This book is written with the *Misophonia Matters* approach at its forefront and includes numerous worksheets and coping tips throughout.

In many ways, this book is a spiritual successor to my 2015 book *Full of Sound and Fury: Living with Misophonia*. Some sections were even repurposed and re-written. This book is a mix of new writing, pieces taken from past articles and perspectives, including excerpts from my 2024 book *Misophonia Matters*, and includes personal stories from myself and other members of the community, and more. The purpose of this book is to provide an overview of misophonia and coping skills for a general public audience. If you would like a more clinical overview of misophonia, as I said above, I recommend checking out *Misophonia Matters* as this provides a more in-depth overview on psychoeducation, sensory regulation, and cognitive-based strategies for coping. I have used most of the worksheets from *Misophonia Matters* throughout this book, as I feel they are useful coping skills tools, and I wanted to ensure that you had access to these.

Any articles and blog posts which have been re-used in this book were done so with intent. It is my hope that reproducing these pieces and re-writing them in places will provide a wide array of topics and ideas which I have been cultivating since the beginning of my advocacy, and now clinical, journey. It is my hope that this book will offer practical coping skills for misophonia, as well as my own perspective on the disorder. This book should in no way replace a clinician, and I highly recommend finding counselling if you feel you need it. The

International Misophonia Foundation offers a provider directory at misophoniafoundation.com/clinicians for you to find a clinician who understands misophonia.

I HAVE MISOPHONIA

At nineteen years old, I lost my ability to fully take part in the world around me. Unlike common sensory impairments, I did not lose my ability to hear, or smell, or see. Instead, I suffer from a condition that amplifies each of these. When I touch, when I look, I am feeling everything around me—and it does not feel pleasant. Imagine you are trapped with the same sound for hours. A slow torture will begin to encapsulate your body. For sufferers of misophonia, a strange yet real condition, this torture is immediate. From the drop of a fork, or the slight pitch of a whistle, we are derailed.

Those that have not heard of misophonia are often surprised by the condition. Some are perplexed by its nature and have trouble believing that it's more than an annoyance. For sufferers of misophonia, we are confronted with an immediate fight/flight/freeze response to otherwise normal sounds and visuals.

When I first discovered my condition, I went through a lot of emotions. The first was relief that I was not crazy. This was quickly followed by dismay. While I did have a name for the disorder, there was no cure. Soon, my dismay turned to frustration. Information on my disorder, when spread, was often wrong, or even blatantly manipulative. Charlatans were capitalizing off Google and Wikipedia, while the editors at sites as big as WebMD weren't paying attention to scientists. I spent the first year of this disorder wondering what would come of everything—if there was no cure, and no one was paying attention, I didn't know how I was supposed to keep going.

Advocating for an unknown condition is multifaceted. For some, my story has become a beacon, and my efforts are a force to be reckoned with. To many, I have become a symbol of hope. I often feel shame when I sit in my worst moments, void of promise and inspiration. While others look up to me, I spend many moments lost in my own dreariness. The truth is that I am uncomfortable with any idolization for my actions. I am an advocate not for notoriety, but for the ultimate end goal. I am an advocate because I hope for a world that people like me can walk freely upon the streets or have dinner in a restaurant.

While stigma is still a problem for many disorders, I have never had as hard of a time as I do with my disorder that is completely unknown. If I must explain my OCD, Anxiety, or Depression to others, I can point them to research studies—to evidence and proof that these disorders are real. For misophonia, these studies are happening, but at a slow pace, and while there is no treatment, research has picked up significantly in the last ten years.

I don't mind being an advocate for my disorder. It's invigorating to know that my day-to-day work may have an impact on my own life and that of current and future sufferers. However, that does not mean I am not tired. I am tired of typing, and saying, the same sentences over and over. I am tired of having to justify my disorder whenever I meet a new person. I am tired of explaining why I cannot go to restaurants, or why jingling keys, tapping hands, or whistling turn me into a nightmare—crying and all. When I first discovered what "misophonia" was, I had an entirely different story to tell. I was scared that I had a disorder that seemed to be under-researched and would be at risk of being stigmatized.

Most people that I have talked to who have misophonia have been suffering since they were children. However, I am one of the late bloomers. Regardless of when it came to be, misophonia is an extremely isolating disorder. I was 16 when I showed my first symptoms, but they were mild. It wasn't until 19 when the full force of misophonia hit me like a freight train. Since then, I have felt its wrath clasp around my throat, taking over several aspects of my life. My first blog post on misophonia was written before I even knew there was a name and before I had anything to go on. I remember writing in frustration, tears not far off, as I wondered why I was so messed up. Why, all of a sudden, I was having so much trouble with sights and sounds? When I first came across misophonia, I described it as ruining my life. I didn't understand why, but these everyday movements and sounds were turning normal situations into a terrible prison. I also wasn't sure if I had this thing called *misophonia* because they were describing an aversion to *sounds* and my visual triggers were just as prominent.

I attributed my first triggers to an anxiety disorder as well as major depressive disorder. Small movements or rocking back and forth were enough to cause near panic attacks. If a desk was not sitting on the floor properly, I would lose it. If a classmate was making loud and distracting noises, I'd complain to the teacher. It didn't always get me far, but if they didn't help, I'd leave. I wasn't the most attentive student in high school.

On January 27th, 2014, I wrote a post expressing my confusion and rage regarding what I now know as misophonia. Please bear in mind that this was written before I had any idea of what misophonia was. The title was "I don't know what to do." Below, it is recopied in full. This is probably my most raw piece on misophonia.

When I first came to university, I didn't remember why I had been so distracted and annoyed in high school. Homework isn't hard, the reading is fine. What I can't deal with is the burden that my anxiety can be in a classroom environment. Half of the time I have a scowl on my face in class and probably come off as a bit of a condescending witch. Whenever people whistle, click their pen, or shake their legs, it's extremely distracting for me and for a reason I cannot explain it sends me into a horrible state. Leg twitching in my peripheral vision has literally brought me to tears. I'm so frustrated that I can't just "get over it". I understand restless leg syndrome is a real thing but so is the anxiety that I suffer every time I enter a classroom. I understand that it would be rude to approach somebody and ask them to please stop torturing me.

Instead, I often stew and try not to get upset but instead I usually just end up irrationally angry. Oftentimes I can actually feel the vibrations on the floor from people shaking behind me, even if they're far away. A couple of weeks ago I started hyperventilating when somebody was whistling. Why? The sharp noise was so unbearable to me. I honestly don't know what I'm supposed to do about this. Breathing exercises, telling myself it's out of my control, and "thinking positive" are hopeless. I don't want to constantly glare at my friends like they're the worst thing in the world just because they're shaking their feet. I'm actually sorry it bugs me this much, but I can't stop. Sometimes I find myself sitting in my room anxious about going to class just because of my triggers. I just feel alone in this and that I must sound ridiculous to others. Aside from hiding in my room wearing earplugs and only ever communicating via Skype I'm not sure of a fix to this.

Misophonia Worksheets

Throughout this book you will find misophonia worksheets for people with misophonia, parents, and couples with misophonia. These worksheets are meant to be used whenever you feel they're necessary, or you can do them as you read along!

My first "real" trigger was whistling. I would go into a rage and nearly cry whenever faced with it. Some people would whistle on purpose, because they did not understand the severity of my reaction. I remember being upset for hours after this would happen, and that confused me a lot. My mother's foot-shaking really started to bother me. Soon after, the sound of singing and country music really sent me over the edge. This caused a lot of fights and confusion. Why was I so intolerant? It made no sense to me.

While there are many triggers that seem to pop up in numerous people, not everybody has the same triggers. We're not all the same, so that makes it even harder to raise awareness. However, regardless of what a person is triggered by, we're still triggered, and it can be very disorienting. There also seems to be a list of triggers that many people have. While some have all of the triggers, others have only a few. I will list these in another chapter.

WHAT EXACTLY IS MISOPHONIA?

If you or a loved one can't stand the sound of chewing, pen-clicking, or whistling, you may have a newly discovered disorder called *misophonia*. The name misophonia comes from the words *miso (hate)* and *phonia (sound)* in Latin. The loose translation for the disorder is *hatred of sound*. This name is a bit simplistic, but it does focus on the distress that sounds causes in the lives of people with misophonia. While this book is written in the perspective of the *disorder* misophonia, it is really about all sound sensitivity, as well as visual stimuli. The heart of this book is about coping with a world that *isn't right for your brain*. It is my hope that whether you believe you have full blown-misophonia (whatever that means) or simply struggle with certain sounds (or visuals), that you will find this book helpful.

I became interested in writing about misophonia for the reason that most others have, wherein I have struggled with misophonia for many years, and I can personally say that it's hell. I would do anything to make misophonia disappear forever, and that's guided a lot of my professional life. From web designer (in 2013) to master's student and clinician (2024), misophonia has changed the trajectory of my life, because without accommodation and finding more acceptance, life would be even harder than it already is.

I get a bit grossed out whenever I see a media-person, talk-show host, or even a clinician, type or say the words, "Is misophonia real?". To me, this feels like a strange question. Why would somebody make up a disorder that causes so much distress? To some, like those who believe everything we do is some kind of behaviour-based conspiracy, maybe they really do believe we want to control the home through the dinner fork. Scientifically speaking, there have been numerous studies in the past 10 years that show that misophonia is in fact a real disorder! There was a Delphi study in 2022 (Swedo) that confirmed this, as well as a 2018 literature review (Brout)—and numerous other studies. I highly suggest you check out the references at the back of this book.

Some people around the community have been calling it "mee-so-phonia" or "m-eye-sophonia". I can see why people would jump to this conclusion, since after all, miso soup is a delicacy in many parts of the world, but *we're not soup*. I could wager that we're not hatred either, but this isn't about what we are, it's about how to pronounce the word.

Dictionary.com defines miso (of Greek origin) as "indicating hatred", but more importantly, it shows another word that starts with the same prefix. Like misogynist, misophonia starts with the Greek word "miso".

With that in mind, I pronounce it relatively the same, as "miss-o-phonia". So, unlike the Japanese word (miso) pronounced "meeso", "miso" is generally pronounced more like misogyny.

Many people ask the question, "Is misophonia psychological?" While the answer to this question is largely based on a small body of research, the answer is nonetheless important. This question is particularly challenging not because of misophonia, but because of the ever-changing field of research and theory. In modern times, it has become increasingly difficult to categorize disorders in this way because disorders overlap, and exact causes often remain unknown. This, of course, adds to the confusion.

Compelling evidence has arisen that points misophonia in a different direction. Instead of psychological, the condition may in fact be neurophysiological (Brout, 2021). Not only this, but it also takes part in the center of the brain that regulates fear, the limbic system. As explorations continue, it seems less likely that misophonia is merely a psychological predicament. However, this does not mean that a cross-disciplinary approach will not be beneficial for the eventual treatment of the disorder.

Miren Edelstein, researcher and author of "Misophonia: physiological investigations and case descriptions" advocates for better communication in the research world, particularly for brain conditions:

> *"I think it would be extremely beneficial to have neuroscientists and audiologists, as well as clinical psychologists, psychiatrists, and physicians, all collaborating together to conduct Misophonia research. Right now, a major problem for Misophonia research that needs to be addressed is the lack of communication between various fields of study. Researchers from different disciplines all have unique and valuable perspectives on the topic, but this information is not being communicated in an effective manner across groups. I believe that an interdisciplinary research environment, while simultaneously promoting a more unified dissemination of knowledge, will be the most effective at fostering breakthroughs in the field."*

The complexity of misophonia is important. While the disorder does have some psychological symptoms, it does not entirely pertain to psychological processes: "In addition to reporting psychological symptoms, all of our misophonics reported physical symptoms synonymous with autonomic arousal in response to trigger sounds" (Edelstein).

While an exact answer on whether or not misophonia is psychological is not yet possible, there is great cause for concern when the condition is mindlessly labelled as psychological. While there is no research yet to confirm that *misophonia* is part of a wider sensory landscape, if it is, I would suggest that we are looking more at *multisensory dysregulation* or *multisensory overload* than we are simply at a "hatred of sound".

IS MISOKINESIA THE SAME AS MISOPHONIA?

One question I am asked occasionally is "how do visual triggers relate to misophonia?" and while that's a great question, and one I wish I knew the answer to, it's unfortunately one that we do not know. In 2014, Schröder proposed the term misokinesia for visual triggers that were present in patients that had misophonia. This term was not meant to coin a new disorder, but more to explain a phenomenon that was not encapsulated by the disorder as it was known at the time.

We do not yet know if all persons with misophonia also have misokinesia (i.e. they are the same disorder), or if some persons with aversive reactions to sound (Misophonia) do not have an aversion to visuals (Misokinesia). It is possible that these aversions happen on a spectrum and are different in each clinical case. This is something that has not yet been researched.

At this time, however, what I can say is that many in the community (myself included) have both visual and auditory triggers that manifest with a similar fight-flight-freeze reaction. For those that do have misokinesia, there is little difference between the nature of the trigger after the outset. Our fight-flight-freeze systems are engaged, we feel discomfort, sometimes pain, and then negative emotional effects.

The term "misophonia" is not the greatest anyways, since we do not "hate" sounds (or visuals), but we are merely experiencing aversive reactions to the way our brains are processing these stimuli as a threat. Yet, this is the name that the popular press and research have clung to and landed upon, so we must accept it for now. In the meantime, it is important to realize that much of the knowledge that we have on both auditory and visual triggers is in the beginning stages of discovery, and nothing is set in stone. While I use the terms misophonia and misokinesia often, I am not married to these terms and do believe we are looking at more of a multisensory overload.

I'd like to first start by saying that misokinesia (hatred of movement) is a term that oversimplifies things. Research-wise, there's not enough to go on to say whether or not visual triggers are different from misophonia. They might both be related, they could be part of a wider sensory dysregulation, or they could be two interlinked disorders. The research simply isn't there. We also don't know whether or not *all*, *most*, or *some* sufferers also have visual triggers. For these purposes, I am just going to use "visual triggers" or "visual stimuli".

My visual triggers are just as hard to handle as my auditory triggers. Sometimes they are worse. I find it nearly impossible to escape a sight in a room. Even when I close my eyes, and even hours or days later, the memory is still there. I want to cry as I think of these triggers. Legs shaking, people swaying, fingers and toes tapping. Even improper grammar has been known to become triggering. Double spacing after periods is so intensely anguished that I've had to block people from communication.

I've had people that have misophonia tell me that "You can't have visual triggers or be triggered by grammar". This has been frustrating, as I fight tooth and nail for advocacy, to be told by my own community that I am "wrong". Having severe visual *and* audial triggers has made life more challenging. The grammar and typing and light effect triggers are so severe that I find it nearly impossible to surf the web or play video games.

For me, visual triggers have been harder to explain because even our own media doesn't do enough to explain. Of course, I can't fault us as there simply isn't enough data (scientific or otherwise). Sometimes it's hard to handle visual triggers because I can't wear earplugs for my eyes. I suppose I could wear a blindfold, but this has impractical implications. I am also more likely to remember visual triggers, and if I have been visually triggered somewhere in the past, I will not want to go back to the place.

I have had dreams of these triggers. I have had waking nightmares. These visuals are so deeply intertwined in my brain that they haunt me like a ghost. Sounds might go away... but the visuals remain. I have stopped having text conversations with many people because they don't understand. I get it, but it's hard for me to socialize. It's become further isolation atop of my isolation. I'm not sure what the answer is, but one thing is for sure, we need more research. This of course is only *my experience* with visual triggers.

Misophonia Worksheet

REASONABLE VERSUS UNREASONABLE REQUESTS

Perhaps one of the hardest parts of misophonia is deciding which triggers should or should not be accommodated by another person. In practice, this is a constant negotiation. This chart is meant to be filled out together with your partner. If you and your partner cannot agree if a request is reasonable or unreasonable, then this is an area for further negotiations and discussions around that particular trigger.

Reasonable Request	Unreasonable Request

COMMON MISOPHONIA TRIGGERS

If you do not wish to read a list of triggers, please feel free to skip this chapter entirely. This chapter is provided as a guide on triggers which have been reported in the literature (Schroder, 2013; Erfanian, 2016; Brout, 2018; Swedo, 2022) but should not be taken as an all-encompassing list. Variability is to be expected, and some people have more triggers than others. You might even have a trigger not listed. I am including visual triggers in the same chapter as auditory chapters for simplicity. However, it should be noted that the relationship between visual and auditory triggers has not been thoroughly researched.

AUDITORY TRIGGERS

Whistling

Chewing

Tapping

Sneezing

Coughing

Snoring

Lawnmowers/leaf blowers

Clicking mouse

Keyboard typing

Pen clicking

Water pouring into a glass

Tongue clicking

Sniffling

Licking sounds

Slurping sounds

Flipflops clacking

Clock ticking

Scraping

Barking

Owl hooting

Birds chirping

Plastic rustling

Styrofoam rubbing

VISUAL TRIGGERS

Leg jiggling/shaking

Foot tapping

Chewing (without sound)

Two spaces after a period

Text speech (u, r, ur)

Blinking text cursor

Flashing lights

An overabundance of punctuation, especially "!"

Untied shoelaces

Effects in video games

Bright lights

Pinwheels, windmills, and all other "rotating" circles

Bags swinging

IS MISOPHONIA MENTAL ILLNESS?

The important question to ask when deciding the misophonia mental illness debate is to define, at least quickly, what a mental illness is, because a lot of people are unsure what constitutes mental illness. There is a general consensus within the medical and advocacy communities that mental illnesses are psychiatric and psychological in nature. According to the American Psychiatric Association, mental illness:

- refers collectively to all diagnosable mental disorders — health conditions involving
- Significant changes in thinking, emotion, and/or behavior
- Distress and/or problems functioning in social, work, or family activities

In my opinion, misophonia is probably not psychiatric. When research isn't conducted to properly find what causes a condition, psychiatry can be quick to slap a label on the condition. In an article in the NY Observer, Dr. Jennifer Brout discusses her conversations with psychiatrists who were "hell-bent" on labeling, diagnosing, and essentially "treating" misophonia:

"I asked the author of many of these studies why he and his colleagues were doing therapy for misophonia when there was absolutely no consensus as to what the disorder was (and when none of their therapies had been trialed). During his transparent explanation, he slipped up and referred to misophonia sufferers as potential "consumers"."

So, does this mean misophonia is not a mental illness? Misophonia is most likely to be neurophysiological, but this does not mean that it is not a mental illness. Some researchers have begun to tip the traditional theory of "illness" upside down. There are emerging ideas and evidence that support a new definition of mental illness. While not a mental illness as strictly defined by iron-clad definitions, in the future there may be a thinner line between disorders that have origins in the brain. An academic paper from 2015 talks about this changing perception.

"The results may be taken as a slap in the face to the distinction-abolitionists, yet such individuals might take heart in them in that there is no implicit hierarchy in what emerges as the brain-based hallmark of neurological versus psychiatric conditions; they both involve the functionally interesting parts of the brain, it is just that they are, quite subtly, different." (Anthony S. David, Timothy Nicholson, 2015)

While confusing to some, this has positive implications for the world of research. Under a paradigm that strips away the strictly worded diagnostics codes of the DSM-5, treatment and research can move past set expectations and work together for cross-disciplinary

MISOPHONIA JOURNAL MOMENT: WHAT ARE YOUR TRIGGERS?

I encourage you to use the space on the side of this page to list your own misophonia triggers. If you are a parent or a loved one, feel free to write their triggers.

_____
_____
_____
_____
_____
_____
_____
_____
_____
_____
_____
_____
_____
_____
_____
_____
_____
_____
_____
_____
_____
_____
_____

approaches. The IMF has advocated for this approach to research. Whether or not misophonia is a mental illness depends upon who you ask. Its basic components are in the brain, more specifically the limbic system. As classifications of disorders continue to change, we may find the definition of mental illness itself will be put into question. However, for now, misophonia is not a mental illness in the sense that it is a diagnosable mental disorder, and in fact, sufferers may have trouble obtaining a misophonia diagnosis at all.

Whether or not a condition is a *mental illness* does not change the fact that there are mental and emotional consequences to the disorder. Even if misophonia is entirely within physical structures of the brain, the lives of sufferers are impacted in ways that have cognitive and emotional impact. Consider a physical condition like epilepsy. The person with this condition might have numerous feelings about their disorder and its impact on their quality of life, even though epilepsy itself is not a *mental illness*. At the end of the day, improving quality of life for those with misophonia is paramount.

LEARNING ABOUT MISOPHONIA

Rather than our thoughts and emotions controlling our physical and emotional reactions to sensory stimuli, the sensory stimuli and fight-flight-freeze reaction are causing the response. A person with misophonia will hear a sound, and then the brain (amygdala) will conceive this sound as a threat which leads to an emotional (and physiological) response. This is why no amount of "thinking the trigger away" will work; your thought process is not coming into the conversation with your brain until *after* you have been triggered by whatever stimuli is causing the misophonic reaction. Why these sounds are triggering a fight-flight-freeze reaction has not yet been discovered.

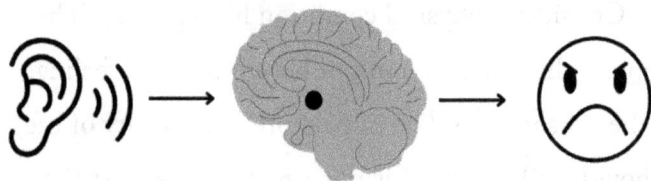

When we stop to think about *why* we are having an emotional reaction, most people do not initially have stories that go alongside triggers. For example, the *first time* we are triggered by something is likely not something that we remember. We may, however, have negative associations of these triggers and times when we were triggered by family and friends—or even specific locations where we were triggered. The emotion, however, comes later than the initial fight-flight-freeze response.

FIGHT, FLIGHT, FREEZE

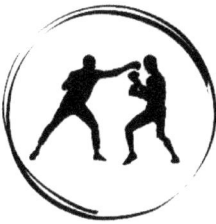 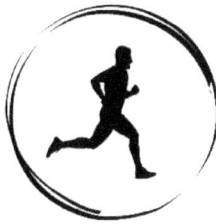 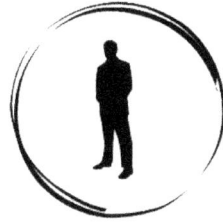

FIGHT   **FLIGHT**   **FREEZE**

When the brain and body enter fight-flight-freeze, there are only three responses available to us as a reaction. We can either fight, flee, or freeze in response. For misophonia, fight rarely amounts to violence unless in young children, yet there might be thoughts of anger and disgust, or a verbal outburst asking the person to stop (perhaps unkindly). Flight is self-explanatory, since when facing triggers, many with misophonia leave the environment if they can. Freeze tends to be more perplexing for those who are triggered and those around them. Freeze can amount to feeling unable to react or even staring at the triggering offender. Consider this, if you were in the room with a person, you do not know who is wielding a knife in your direction—would you take your eyes off the knife?

Fight-flight-freeze is our body's way of helping us identify and deal with threats, and for reasons we do not yet know, misophonia causes this release of adrenaline in the body which causes distress after hearing a trigger sound. Habituation refers to the state where a person becomes accustomed to a state or stimuli. For people with misophonia, habituation is a state that we never achieve as our nervous systems do not become accustomed to the triggering sounds or visuals. This is also why exposure therapy is inappropriate.

WHAT IS THE AUTONOMIC NERVOUS SYSTEM?

The Autonomic Nervous System (ANS) is a complex part of the body that controls the fight-flight-freeze response, as well as other necessary functions for human existence:

"The autonomic nervous system is a component of the peripheral nervous system that regulates involuntary physiologic processes including heart rate, blood pressure, respiration, digestion, and

sexual arousal. It contains three anatomically distinct divisions: sympathetic, parasympathetic, and enteric" (Waxenbaum, 2023)

This is a complex system of the body that has many functions necessary for survival.

"The autonomic nervous system (ANS) is made up of pathways of neurons that control various organ systems inside the body, using many diverse chemicals and signals to maintain homeostasis. It divides into the sympathetic and parasympathetic systems. The sympathetic component is better known as "fight or flight" and the parasympathetic component as "rest and digest." It functions without conscious control throughout the lifespan of an organism to control cardiac muscle, smooth muscle, and exocrine and endocrine glands, which in turn regulate blood pressure, urination, bowel movements, and thermoregulation" (LeBouef, 2023)

The sympathetic part of the autonomic nervous system is responsible for the fight-flight-freeze system, whereas the parasympathetic part is responsible for stopping the fight-flight-freeze response. The fight-flight-freeze response is first detected by the amygdala, which then alerts the hippocampus to activate the sympathetic nervous system. Once this is activated, adrenaline rushes through the system, elevates the heartrate, and causes what people describe as the "anxious" response. The parasympathetic system is responsible for stopping this response and thus helps the body reach what many refer to as "calm". The enteric system deals with digestion and will not be touched upon in this book, although I suspect there are more complexities involving multisensory dysregulation and the digestive system.

While we know that people with misophonia are having a fight-flight-freeze response, we do not know *why* this is happening. More rigorous research and brain-based studies will be necessary to fully decipher the origins of misophonia and its reasons for onset. While the nervous system is an important component for understanding misophonia, it can be helpful to avoid getting lost in the weeds of complicated neurophysiological processes, especially given the preliminary status of this research. However, if one is interested in reading more about the brain basis for misophonia, the best place to start is this study by Dr. Sukhbinder Kumar:

Kumar, S., Tansley-Hancock, O., Sedley, W., Winston, J.S., Callaghan, M.F., Allen, M., Cope, T.E., Gander, P.E., Bamiou, D.E., & Griffiths, T.D. (2017). The brain basis for misophonia. *Current Biology, 27*(4).

https://www.sciencedirect.com/science/article/pii/S09609
82216315305?via%3Dihub

WHAT IF YOUR DOCTOR HASN'T HEARD OF MISOPHONIA

If your doctor has never heard of misophonia, it is harder to obtain care. Unfortunately, misophonia is a lesser-known condition so few doctors and medical professionals have hands-on experience with the disorder. While your doctor is a trained healthcare professional, they are not psychic. This means that fields are ever-changing, and there is a reason it is called medical *practice*. If your doctor has not heard of misophonia, it is okay to teach them about the disorder. In fact, self advocacy is a reliable tool for taking your health seriously.

Medical professionals that are reliable should be compassionate to your condition. If they are not, this leaves concern for the quality of care. While a doctor, psychologist, audiologist, or neurologist may not know what misophonia is, it is important that they are willing to listen to the patient's symptoms and feelings and understand that this condition is having an impact on the patient's life. Professionals should be willing to work in a cross-disciplinary capacity and should be willing to become educated on preliminary research of the condition.

While there is no official cure, a doctor (or medical professional) can help you learn to cope with the disorder. Until research is furthered, professionals can work across fields to come up with cognitive and physiological strategies that benefit the patient. Occupational therapists that have worked with sensory integration and processing cases may be well equipped to understand the nuances of misophonia in a sensory capacity.

In an article for the Huffington Post, I shared "What I Wish My Doctor Knew About Misophonia". In this piece, I penned a letter for my doctor, explaining that while I understood they were unable to cure my condition, I needed support on my medical journey. This was mailed to my primary care physician who has been nothing but supportive of my misophonia journey. While there is no official diagnosis available, I am confident that my doctor listens to my needs.

I want my doctor to know that if he acknowledges my suffering and asks me how I think we should go about things, that he is doing what he can. I want him to know that I do not expect miracles; I merely expect his patience. I want my doctor to know that if he does not know about my disorder, that is okay. I want him to know that I will be happy to work with him on this discovery.

If your doctor has not heard of misophonia and is unwilling to learn, then it is perhaps best to look at your options for finding a primary care physician that is willing to think of your needs. Not every doctor will be a good fit.

DO YOUR SENSES MAKE SENSE TO YOU?

In primary school, we quickly learn that we have five senses. This knowledge is no longer scientifically accurate, and yet much of the public has never heard of the other three senses that make up our more complete eight-sense system. Researchers of autism and sensory integration have come a long way at studying the human body and have classified the eight senses as the following: sight, olfactory (scent), hearing, touch (tactile), taste, interoception (knowledge of what is going on in our body), proprioception (sense of movement and location), and vestibular (sense of balance). Research on misophonia shows that the interoception sense is involved in misophonia as well as the auditory sense (Kumar, 2017). Early research on misophonia has shown that the disorder is far more complicated than simply hearing a sound and getting angry or distressed.

WHAT IS SENSORY-REGULATION AND SELF-REGULATION?

Sensory regulation is "the ability to select and process sensory information to plan and perform appropriate behaviors" (Piccardi and Gliga, 2022). Rather than our behavior being something that is driven by our cognitive needs, it is instead driven by our neurophysiological and sensory needs (Dunn, 2014). Self-regulation refers to the ability to manage our own physiological states and choose behaviors in accordance with these states (Shanker and Barker, 2016). For the purpose of this book, when I mention "sensory regulation", I am referring to the ability to calm the nervous system when triggered by sensory stimuli.

LIVING WITH MISOPHONIA ISN'T EASY

One thing that I want to impress upon readers, whether they have misophonia or know someone who does, is that the disorder is not easy to live with. Being constantly bombarded by complex fight-flight-freeze reactions is unnatural, and the panic can become increasingly related to a fear of having triggers, not just the trigger moment. When you consider how unpleasant misophonia is, there should be no surprise that avoidance and fear are often associated with an increased exposure risk. I have yet to find a person with misophonia who isn't worried about the *next* time they'll be triggered, often associating past experiences with the risk of future triggering environments. Safety becomes of absolute concern when you're worried about the pain and discomfort of triggers.

As a person with misophonia, I spend a lot of my time worried about the next time I'll be triggered. While this is not behavior that serves me, it is completely rational to worry about future pain. That said, there needs to be a balance where one can live their life with misophonia, and much of this comes from reducing the panic surrounding the trigger moment—these moments where there is no stimuli present, and yet we're still on edge. These are the moments that we can take back and learn to live around misophonia, rather than cowering from its ever-imposing presence.

Learning to live around this moment is not without its bitterness; there are times where I wish I didn't have to constantly debate if an experience is worth the risk, or that I could simply venture into my backyard without worry. And yet, this is not the reality I live in, and thus I must adapt to the circumstances. I am aware that this is not *fair*, and yet, it is the harsh truth that each of us with this disorder must confront; especially as there is currently no treatment for the disorder that can remediate all symptoms. So, what now?

As I present in *Misophonia Matters*, my approach to coping with misophonia is three-pronged and involves advocacy, sensory regulation, and cognitive and psychological skills. Advocacy can be as simple as presenting your condition to those in your life and asking for accommodation. Sensory regulation involves the use of a sensory diet which has been the main tool of occupational therapists for Sensory Integration, Autism, and Sensory Processing Disorder. Cognitive and Psychological tools then help us to reconcile with our beliefs surrounding misophonia and learn how to adapt and live with the reality of our situation.

EXPOSURE THERAPY DOES NOT WORK

While speaking in confidence with me, many individuals with misophonia have expressed their horrific experiences with exposure therapy in research or clinical environments. Parents of children with misophonia have reached out with concerns that these practices seemed cruel and unreasonable when used on their children. So, why do practitioners, particularly those who cling to a CBT model, still continue to use this practice? Small-scale studies on misophonia are often used as a justification for CBT by showing in non-replicable results that these studies "worked". There is often no follow-up other than a brief survey seeing if the treatment worked immediately after.

What I propose is happening is that many people with misophonia might be reacting to these studies first with a placebo effect. For some with misophonia, before this 'researcher' or 'clinician' has attempted to treat their misophonia, they may have never been validated as having a real condition. As I have done surveys/research that has not been published yet (but will be within the next year), many sufferers of misophonia note the following cognitive dissonance: a) their misophonia was not treated by the intervention of exposure therapy (or even CBT), and b) they did not tell the practitioner this did not work, and there was no follow-up asking them to do so at intervals. These persons often tell me that they were grateful for the help, and report strong feelings of positive regard for practitioners, whilst also believing that the treatment was either not beneficial, or in some cases, even made them feel worse.

As I have repeated for years, if exposure therapy worked, then we would all be cured. There is not a day on earth where persons with misophonia are not triggered. These sounds are everyday persistent sounds which we are never able to escape. We are not simply afraid of these sounds—it is not a cognitive-based fear. For example, I will wake up from a dead sleep if there is a trigger present. This is not a manifested or learned response. We are feeling these sounds at a much deeper brain level, which has been proven in far better research than what has been presented by any CBT therapist.

I have absolutely no idea why so many practitioners are so obsessed with the idea of exposure therapy. Imagine being so arrogant that you ignore the voices of those with the disorder telling you something does not work. I have yet to meet an actual person with misophonia (researcher, clinician, general public) who will say exposure therapy works. Why not? Because it doesn't. How often do I have to tell practitioners to stop doing exposure therapy? At this point, it feels like for the rest of my life.

As a sidenote, not all CBT is misophonia, and CBT can be helpful in many ways in our lives. That is completely different than exposure therapy, which is absolutely not the answer to misophonia.

Clinicians and researchers of those with misophonia must be weary and aware of their very real power imbalance in these studies. Many persons with misophonia have been ignored, mistreated, or simply told that their disorder does not exist. The mere presence of a clinician telling them that misophonia is real, is in itself a powerful motivator to not tell the clinician that they were not helped. Often, I have been told by persons with misophonia that they believed the treatment would work on another person, but felt they were just "too crazy" or "too broken to be fixed". I have also been told that these participants felt like they did not want to let down or make their clinician/researcher who tried so hard to help them feel better, so they said that it worked to spare their feelings. This, of course, is something that the clinicians should have been aware of and worked to keep out of their studies. And yet, this phenomenon persists, and the research is tainted by its very design.

If misophonia could be treated by exposure therapy, every single blog, advocate, and person with misophonia would be crying with relief and screaming from the rooftops. As a clinician, advocate, and person with misophonia, I will tell you that there are absolutely no accounts that I can see of a person with misophonia who has, in fact, been "cured" by exposure therapy. There are, however, (and sadly), hundreds who have told me that exposure therapy caused them PTSD and ruined their lives.

MISOPHONIA IS NOT A LIFE SENTENCE

There's no question that misophonia changes the lives of those who suffer from it. It also changes the lives of parents, siblings, friends, and romantic partners. This doesn't mean that you need to hide your entire life. Sure, it's hard to live with, but life is still possible with these complications. With a few adjustments, you can have a normal, fulfilling life.

You may have to change what your idea of "normal" is to match your needs. After all, life is about what you make it. Stop thinking of misophonia as something that has "happened to you" and start thinking about it as an interesting part of you. I know that can be hard to consider. After all, it sucks. But, think of it this way, this is a part of who you are for better or worse.

Figuring out what can help with misophonia in the 2020s is a landmine. A quick world wide web search for "treatments for misophonia" will land you thousands of results—some of which are asking for payments for apps, hypnotherapy, or other promised treatments. One time I even found an essential oil blend which *literally claimed to cure misophonia*. I was shocked and horrified… but a small part of me also laughed at the absurdity. There are some options that do offer some help for the condition, but wading through the depths of charlatans to land on a helpful coping skill or treatment becomes unlikely when we consider that Google does not regulate advertisements for treatments, and thus, anybody can pay to serve you advertisements regardless of the ethics.

Tangent aside, coping with misophonia is something that varies from person to person. Each person with misophonia has different variations of triggers, different needs for things that they are unable to live without, such as eating dinner with a loved one, and different ideas and opinions on how misophonia impacts their life. This variability does not mean that nothing can help misophonia, but it does mean that any person seeking self-help must consider their own needs specifically.

Part of dealing with the variability of misophonia, at least in my opinion, is developing communication and negotiation skills by way of advocating for yourself or a loved one with misophonia. Through this process we can move through the world of misophonia and our sensory needs by learning how to adapt and negotiate our way through these uncomfortable moments. For example, no amount of deep breathing exercise will help me to sit in a room with a clicking pen.

What could happen is a negotiation that allowed me to avoid sitting in the room in the first place, or the ability to wear earplugs or a sound generator in this room. I will still have misophonia, but I will be able to mitigate this fight-flight-freeze response through a reasonable accommodation which is achieved through advocacy.

It is my firm belief that coping with misophonia is a work of advocacy. In fact, managing most disorders whether neurological, neurophysiological, or psychological requires a degree of advocacy to help cope with the disorder and navigate a world that is not built for your brain chemistry. Advocacy can be as simple as negotiating with a loved one how you will manage your home lives with your condition, or as complex as engaging in public awareness, writing letters, and influencing policy that impacts misophonia. There is no level of advocacy, however, that is required for misophonia by default. Your own level of comfort should dictate the level you engage in advocacy. There is no right or wrong!

Before we discuss potential coping skills for misophonia, I think it is important to mention that any life change that you make that helps you cope with misophonia is your own form of coping skill, and so long as it is not maladaptive and harmful, this is a meaningful state of change.

One way to cope is by masking sounds. For misophonia, I often use pink noise (specifically, the sound of mountain rain) as I personally find it the least jarring of noises. Since there is no actual research on the noises of misophonia and why each sound is a trigger, we do not really know enough to say which noise will be most beneficial. I personally prefer a pink noise, but others might do better with brown or white. The research on sound masking is an ever-developing field with little research in general, and none to date on misophonia. The most important part of these sound masking types is that you personally feel calmed and soothed by it. You can even use a combination at different times and find what works for you specifically.

I personally like to combine pink noise with ear plugs. I find that the combination of both blocks most triggers, whilst it also gives me protection from the white noise being too loud and damaging my ears. Noise-cancelling headphones paired with earplugs can work in public. At home, I play pink noise through my speakers in my room as I find wearing earplugs and headphones continuously can give me a headache. While you can purchase devices specifically to play these sounds, Spotify, Amazon Music, and other music stores often have files that you can play on your mobile devices or speakers.

Many people I see (especially parents) worry that misophonia will get worse as a person ages. However, I want to come and tell you that there is no evidence that this is true. In fact, most people seem to stick with the same triggers they have (there are about twenty of them that are common: whistling, chewing, coughing, snoring, etc.).

Misophonia, instead of getting better or worse over time, "waxes and wanes" (Brout, 2021). What this means is that there are times when a person is more troubled by sounds, whilst during other times they can handle them better. If you are stressed during exams, a divorce, or any other life event, then it stands to reason that your nervous system and fight-flight-freeze response are going to be completely out of whack too. Similarly, during uplifting life events, misophonia can be on the backburner. For example, I remember misophonia being less of a concern whilst completely in bliss after my partner said "I love you" for the first time. It was an opportune moment to go to a movie theatre (and I think we actually did).

Similarly, avoidance is not going to make triggers better or worse. It is completely okay to take your time and stay at home or wear headphones. There is no reason to believe that people are going to make misophonia worse by avoiding triggers. I for one can say that if I take regular breaks and establish boundaries, then my overall happiness level is much greater!

Misophonia Worksheet

THE EMPTY CHAIR

The Empty Chair is a form of Gestalt therapy where the person who is trying to overcome their emotions sits opposite an empty chair and expresses how they feel to the chair. For persons with misophonia, this could be used by either the sufferer of misophonia or by the person who is often causing the triggering sound.

Instructions
- Place an empty chair across from where you are going to sit during this exercise.
- Spend 10 to 20 minutes explaining how you feel to the empty chair. It is best to think of one common theme (such as your chewing popcorn during movies upsets me).
- Take some time to reflect and allow this to sink in. Were you surprised by your feelings?
- Switch your position into the other chair. You are now taking on the role of your partner.
- For 10 to 20 minutes, consider how they feel and express what you think they are feeling. Perhaps the response is "Not being able to enjoy a snack during a movie feels like I am missing out on the experience I am used to."

Reflect on your roleplay as your partner. How did that feel?
This exercise could be used by either partner in the relationship.

MALADAPTIVE VERSUS ADAPTIVE COPING MECHANISMS

People with misophonia and sensory integration issues in general (think autism, sensory processing, etc.) create ways to cope without even thinking about it. Some of these coping methods are adaptive and some of them are maladaptive.

A maladaptive coping mechanism is when we find ways to cope that are counterproductive to the thing we are trying to cope with or otherwise harmful for health. Common maladaptive behaviors are unhealthy foods, cigarettes, drug misuse, alcohol abuse, gambling, and self-harm. This is not an exhaustive list, but rather highlights that maladaptive coping mechanisms are not only unhelpful long-term, but often harmful.

On the other hand, an adaptive coping mechanism is something that is both helpful for misophonia and anxiety and also beneficial for the long-term health of the individual. Common examples of adaptive coping mechanisms are engaging in exercise, yoga, a well-balanced nutritious diet, drinking water, and spending time in nature.

In an audio interview in 2015, Dr. Stephen Porges noted that clients with misophonia often have a higher incidence of maladaptive behaviors (https://www.misophoniainternational.com/the-polyvagal-theory-2/). More research is necessary for confirming this phenomenon, but it is unsurprising to me to think that people with misophonia who never learned how to regulate—or even *what regulation is*—are not gravitating toward adaptive coping skills for misophonia. It is also possible that because misophonia is hardwired so deep in the brain that the person did try traditional adaptive coping mechanisms such as eating right, exercise, and yoga, and were met with a crushing defeat—they still had misophonia, so why bother?

ADAPTION NOT MANIPULATION

For parents of misophonic children, romantic partners, friends, and educators, some traits of misophonia might look to them as manipulative behavior. For those with misophonia, when we are in fight-flight-freeze mode and dysregulated, our brains and bodies are telling us to do *anything* to stop the trigger—just as I imagine one would in any scenario that the brain and body have earmarked as a threat. It should be no surprise that when faced with an extremely aversive reaction to sounds (or visuals), a person with misophonia would go to extreme lengths to stop the noise. Examples of this might include creating alternative explanations to try and force the event not to happen. For example, one might say they cannot go out because they have to do x, y, or z. Perhaps a partner goes to great lengths to avoid date night, even cancelling with excuses. Maybe the person comes up with a story for why something cannot be in their presence—for example, they might respond to gum chewers by saying that they are allergic to the smell. A parent with misophonia may tell their child that their loud chewing is rude, which is socially true in many circumstances, but this might not be the motivation for the request.

On the surface, these behaviors might seem manipulative. The definition of manipulate is to "control or influence a person or situation cleverly, unfairly, or unscrupulously." The key point here is "unfairness" or "unscrupulously". For persons with misophonia, it is not control of the other person that they want to achieve, but rather to alleviate or prevent a misophonic reaction. This behavior is adaptive. People with misophonia are accustomed to being ignored, ridiculed, and told that their condition is not real. Even those who feel supported might deal with guilt for asking others to stop a behavior due to misophonia and thus might rationalize an excuse that is to them more "logical" even if the receiving party suspects that misophonia is the cause. An important part of misophonia is learning to self-advocate and adapt with the condition. However, for some, it can be harder, especially if the other party is not open to learning about their condition or accommodating it. Instead of thinking people with misophonia are manipulative, let us consider that maybe they are just trying to avoid an unpleasant neurophysiological reaction, rather than controlling the person making the trigger for nefarious reasons.

DOES CBT HELP MISOPHONIA?

Many scientists run around telling the world that the "treatment" for misophonia is Cognitive Behavioural Therapy. I think it is important to note that any findings on CBT that have been seen are akin to that of a coping skill—they help deal with the emotional after-effects of misophonia, not the misophonic moment, and certainly not as a preventative measure. You cannot CBT the misophonia away, and you surely should not be out there referring to CBT as a "treatment" for misophonia. This is a disingenuous move by researchers, clinicians, and those involved in the use of CBT to skew public perception on CBT.

I am not saying that CBT is unhelpful for misophonia. Like all coping skills approaches, there is space for CBT in the room when we are trying to help people with misophonia mitigate the after-effects of the disorder and learn how to live in a world that is unaccommodating to their sensory needs. Yet, this does not mean that CBT is the be all and end all, and it absolutely does not mean that we should be toting things like exposure therapy (if exposure worked, we'd all be cured, none of us can completely ignore stimuli). Misophonia is also not a behavioural disorder. We do not *learn* to hate sounds and we cannot *learn not to*. In fact, saying that misophonia is "hatred of sounds" in general is untrue because there is already evidence that there is a brain basis and the amygdala and fight-flight-freeze response are involved (Kumar, 2018).

I understand that scientists are using the language they are used to, but they should be cautious when explaining any cognitive based, or even sensory-based, skill for misophonia as a "treatment". The very word treatment assumes that misophonia can be mitigated by the skills learned, and that is simply not true. CBT is helpful to take the edge off and learn how to understand misophonia through worksheets and psychoeducation, but that does not mean that it should be referred to as a treatment. In-fact, I'd wager that calling anything a treatment at this point in time is nothing more than wishful thinking.

Much of the problem, I assume, is the reliance on "treatments" in American medicine and "psychiatric care". The use of insurance codes means that specific interventions must be referred to as a treatment to be approved for use and reimbursement. Frankly, this entire practice is backwards and wrong and is why in places like Canada where I live this is unheard of and only muddies the waters when it comes to the expectations of those receiving these "treatments". Instead, practitioners and researchers should be honest and explain CBT for what it is, a coping skill for the disorder, and not the be all and end all approach to helping sufferers.

Recently it was pointed out to me by a professional that I respect that my rhetoric on CBT is that of... well... an esteemed hater. I think it's fair to point out that as a person I have been *very* hard on CBT when it comes to misophonia, perhaps zealously. This caused me to pause and reflect, even ever so slightly... on the message that I've been putting out into the world. Now, I will tell you that I am still cautious when it comes to CBT and its use for misophonia, but this mainly applies to exposure therapy.

CBT as a skill is something that is incredibly useful for helping with the *emotional* and *cognitive* effects of misophonia that surround it—this can include social relationships, ideas of self and others, and the distress that follows living a life with misophonia. For that reason, however, I consider CBT to be a coping skill and not a "treatment" in the sense that you will still have misophonia even if you do vigorous CBT. In a way, CBT is almost like a mental health maintenance plan that can help you stay on track and not get lost in the throes of misophonia rage.

In fact, I use CBT for myself and my clients with misophonia regularly. I believe that CBT has a place within the counselling room, and I also believe that it can be used alongside sensory regulation approaches, mindfulness, and other schools of thought like narrative-based therapy. I take a "choose your own adventure" approach to coping with misophonia, however, and I caution practitioners not to stick to an intervention that the client has not responded well to. We're all different! Below are some of the

CHOOSING A MANTRA

Some people with misophonia find choosing a mantra for the misophonic moment to be helpful. The purpose of your mantra should be to both distract yourself from the trigger and remind yourself that you are technically *safe*. For example: "I am safe. This is not forever. I will be okay."
Write your own mantra

_____

_____

_____

_____

_____

_____

_____

_____

_____

_____

_____

_____

types of CBT that I find to be very useful for persons with misophonia.

SMART goals. SMART goals are specific, measurable, achievable, realistic, and time limited.

Guided discovery and questioning. By questioning the assumptions you have about yourself or your current situation, your therapist can help you learn to challenge these thoughts and consider different viewpoints.

Journaling. You might be asked to jot down negative beliefs that come up during the week and the positive ones you can replace them with.

Self-talk. Your therapist may ask what you tell yourself about a certain situation or experience and challenge you to replace negative or critical self-talk with compassionate, constructive self-talk.

Cognitive restructuring. This involves looking at any cognitive distortions affecting your thoughts—such as black-and-white thinking, jumping to conclusions, or catastrophizing—and beginning to unravel them.

Source: https://www.healthline.com/health/cognitive-behavioral-therapy#techniques

I personally believe that most of these have use within misophonia coping skills (albeit some more than others, and obviously never exposure therapy). It is my belief that a practitioner treating misophonia needs to be eclectic and willing to bend their theory and perspective based on the person in front of them—this is even more true with misophonia where we are alleviating symptoms rather than removing the misophonic response.

If the person with misophonia is seeing their quality of life improve from a modality, then that's the right choice, no matter *what* that modality is. I personally like a mix of sensory regulation, CBT, psychodynamic, humanistic, and solution-focused, with some narrative therapy sprinkled in.

Much of my disdain for CBT is not from CBT as a therapy, but rather, the practitioners who are arrogantly proclaiming themselves as "experts in treating misophonia"— to this date I do not think a *single* expert exists, especially since misophonia is such a newly recognized condition. Yet, I think it's important for the record to show that I am not against CBT, and in fact, *Misophonia Matters* includes an entire cognitive section.

DO BEHAVIOURAL ANALYSTS HAVE ANY BUSINESS TREATING MISOPHONIA?

As a new, lesser-known condition, there is one thing I think needs to be verified by scientific efforts so that we can settle the debate once and for all: do behavioural analysts have any business treating misophonia? The most basic answer to this question is that currently, no one has any business treating misophonia. What I find most disturbing is that behavioural analysts have stepped into the fold to try and offer a "remedy" for the condition. Now, there is nothing illegal here so long as they are operating within the confines of their professional industry, but I worry that some of these "behaviour" specialists are toting exposure therapy—which I do not believe works.

I would suggest that currently audiologists, neurologists, psychiatrists, psychologists, and psychotherapists have no official treatment for misophonia, and thus *nobody* should be claiming to offer treatment for the disorder. Behavioural analysts and even cognitive-behavioural-based therapists in my experience have been the most egotistical when saying they have the answers for misophonia. This is, of course, ignoring the verifiable evidence that misophonia has a brain-based component that is deeper than cognitive functions.

It is my opinion that ethically based practices should always be scientifically based. Misophonia is not in any diagnostic manual and yet you can find "providers" who claim they can "cure" and "treat" the disorder. However, I have yet to find actual proof that any of these "treatments" work. Sensory information is cumulative, and many behavioural therapies are essentially torture devices. As I said in 2016, this is in my opinion a cash grab. However, I know I cannot speak for these clinicians and their beliefs and intentions. That said, I can't imagine still toting a treatment despite persons with the disorder, research, and parents of those with the disorder begging for these practices to stop.

Persons with misophonia have the right to choose the services and treatments they want. Practitioners have the right to offer treatments within their scope of practice. But, at what point do we admit that offering "treatments" for a disorder that has not yet seen confirmed treatments in literature or double-blind studies is unethical? I have my doubts that behavioural analysts will provide adequate treatments. By distilling misophonia to a "behaviour" problem, we are furthering the stigma that persons with misophonia are merely bratty children who have just been "raised-wrong" or are trying to control others. We are not. We are people who would do anything in the world to not have this disorder. I am sick of practitioners suggesting otherwise.

GENERAL COPING TIPS

Some of these tips might seem like a "duh" moment, but they are important, nonetheless. I am not suggesting by any means that the following tips will *cure* misophonia, but rather that they will increase quality of life overall, helping us along our path with misophonia by giving us more energy, health, and a lower baseline stress level. With that said, if you do all of these things and are frustrated that your misophonia is still bad, I want to reassure you that you're doing nothing wrong. Each one of us has a different tolerance level, different nervous system, and different level of stress caused by the trigger moment—regardless of other life factors.

LIVING A HEALTHY LIFESTYLE

No matter the disorder, I am a firm believer that a healthy lifestyle is our first line of defense; however, I am perfectly capable of ignoring this advice when stressed, depressed, or just craving endless bread.

I have been struggling with OCD and depression for much of my life, followed by misophonia. Through this journey, I have learned that the most important tool for coping is to understand that we are beings that live lives of connectivity. With that said, I am by no means perfect at following this advice. I eat too many carbs and sugars, I don't exercise enough, and I find it hard to find space to meditate. I say this because I don't want you to think that I believe a *perfect* adherence to health is necessary, but I am merely advocating for doing what we can, when we can. Sleep is probably the one area of health that I am adamant about. I am absolutely useless without sleep, and therefore engage in it luxuriously.

MISOPHONIA JOURNAL MOMENT:

What are some lifestyle changes you could make to lower your everyday stress levels?

List them here.

_____
_____
_____
_____
_____
_____
_____
_____
_____
_____
_____
_____
_____
_____
_____
_____
_____
_____
_____
_____
_____

The following information is mostly my opinion and should be taken with a grain of salt. However, I don't think it is harmful or controversial to say "drink water, sleep, and eat healthily" no matter the condition or lack of evidence on one condition in particular.

WATER INTAKE

It isn't a coincidence that water holds a place at the top of this list. Water is absolutely crucial for a healthy lifestyle. I never knew how dehydrated I was for years until I started drinking an appropriate amount of water. Like a good shower, water has washed away a lot of the cloudiness from my life. Triggers aren't completely alleviated, but I have more energy, I am less stressed, and I feel as though the world is a brighter place. There's never an excuse not to drink enough water, ever. I swear by the practice. In order to make it feasible, I use a free iPhone app called Waterlogged to track how much water I drink daily. I don't always meet my goal, and when I don't, I notice it quickly. The negative aftermath goes well into the next day. The rule I follow is to drink half your weight in ounces.

While some doctors and nutritionists have other ideas, this works for me. I feel so much better now that I drink a good amount of water every day. For example, since I am 150 lbs. right now, I drink at least 75 ounces of water a day. I usually exceed my goal by rounding up to 80 ounces. To make it easier, I measure my water in 20 oz. bottles and then pour it into a glass. Once I'm done with the entire bottle, I register it in the app.

Additionally, I measure my teacups. Each cup of tea is 10 ounces of water. I get a lot of my water from herbal tea which I used to hate. Remember, the feeling of thirst means you're already dehydrated. Drink water at regular intervals throughout the day. You may want to avoid drinking a lot before bedtime as a full bladder can lead to restlessness and an inability to sleep.

You may want more water depending on how you feel, or if you're very active. Listen to your body. If you're unsure about your daily intake, make sure you consult your doctor. Don't be afraid to ask questions that sound odd. It's perfectly reasonable to ask your doctor about your water intake. It's wise, even.

DIET

Misophonia may not be cured by eating right, but a lot of people who suffer from the disorder have noted that they feel much better, and are triggered less, when on a healthy and "clean" diet. High sugar and processed diets aren't doing you any favors. This is especially true if you are already dealing with a condition as strange and discouraging as misophonia. Perhaps eating right won't "cure" misophonia, but eating improperly leads to stress on the body, and when you're stressed, you're more likely to be triggered. I do not advocate for one diet over another, as this is something that is highly controversial, and must be considered on an individual basis that includes scientific research and even cultural factors.

Personally, I feel much better now that I have incorporated a significant number of vegetables, proper protein and reduced sugar, sodium, and processed food intake. It's important to believe that healthy food is not worse, or a punishment. When done right, healthy food is highly rewarding and delicious.

I would never recommend a fad or niche diet. I'm a firm believer in nutrition being a very personal thing. It is not a one size fits all ordeal. Some people are lactose intolerant, but others aren't. I eat milk, cheese and dairy, despite certain warnings. Personally, I have opted for organic options and I feel much better.

Since there is little proof as to what exactly long-term chemical exposure, or even GMOs, are going to do to the body, I believe it is important to be considerate of these factors. That does not mean that you should make choices based on conspiracy theories but simply be aware. You should try different options and see what your body thinks about them. Let your mental and physical health be your guide for what is right for you.

As for cooking, it is an important part of the daily ritual. Much of modern life has become an avoidance of preparation and "busy work." But it is these exact activities that may help us to regulate our sensory systems. As well, preparing your meals yourself gives your body the proper chance it needs to prepare for food and aids digestion.

DOES THE KETOGENIC (KETO) DIET HELP MISOPHONIA?

I have been on the ketogenic diet off and on for a few years, and I wish I could say that suddenly my misophonia had disappeared and that the cure I needed all along had been to simply change my diet, but that is simply not true. While the ketogenic diet has been shown to be helpful for epilepsy (D'Andrea, 2019), we do not know enough about the brain to know whether ketosis is something that can be helpful for misophonia. More importantly, misophonia itself is something that seems to be multi-faceted when it comes to the brain and body (Kumar, 2017).

At this point, I can tell you both from my anecdotal experience and the lack of scientific evidence that the ketogenic diet cannot be considered a treatment for misophonia. Yet, this does not mean that there are no benefits that can be had for persons with misophonia. Importantly, when the body is in distress, misophonia is worse. For those who are obese, have certain food allergies, or feel sluggish due to dietary concerns, finding a diet (any really) that changes their physiological state for the better can reduce the impact of distress after leaving a triggering situation. The better you feel overall, the easier it is to calm down.

Overall health is important for misophonia because we only have one nervous system and one body, and any positive change is beneficial for your long-term coping. That is not to say that the ketogenic diet is the "right" choice, but merely that it is the right choice if a person determines that they have a good experience on the diet. This should always be done with the consultation of a medical professional and dietician, because the diet is such an important tool for health and wellbeing.

For me, dietary choices were more about overall health than misophonia. I haven't noticed my triggers lessened by the diet, but I do have more energy than I did before—which is helpful for an overtaxed nervous system.

EXERCISE

The least fun out of any of these, exercise always seems to land at the bottom of every to-do list. Aside from some gym enthusiasts, exercise is seen as some form of modern torture. I have to admit, I'm not a fan. However, I won't dispute that for some, exercise can provide an amazing high. You don't have to train for a marathon or be an Olympic swim champion to reap the benefits of exercise. Start off slowly. Thirty minutes, three times a week of a physical activity that you enjoy will get the ball rolling, and the more you do, the more you'll feel able and willing to do it. Try to make exercise fun by bringing a friend along. A friend who understands your misophonia and who is willing to compromise will be best. You don't want to be trying to combat triggers while trying to de-stress. However, if you're already triggered, you can use exercise as a way to relieve the tension and beat out the anger. Think boxing.

When I first wrote this section, I was entirely unaware of the proposed benefits of sensory diets used by occupational therapists or the role exercise can play. Since learning this, I have been considering all options and trying things that may help to regulate instead of just picking an exercise and going for it.

I like to choose things like swimming because I feel most comfortable in the water. But I live in Canada so this can be hard in the winter. That's when I enjoy things like bowling, skating, or sledding. I'll admit it's hard to adjust to going out in public and being triggered at first, but when you're bringing along friends and having fun, you may just forget that you're in a "high risk" environment.

MENTAL HEALTH

So many of our emotions are tied to our state of mental health. A good mood can help you to push triggers aside. If you're happy, you're less likely to let a trigger bring you into a state of depression or heightened anxiety. Mental health can bring a trigger from feeling like the apocalypse to feeling like a bump on the knee. This is one way that a therapist can be beneficial. They may not understand misophonia, but they do understand how to help others to live a stress-free life and to make meaningful changes in order to feel happier and more fulfilled, despite any challenges. Co-morbid conditions like OCD, Anxiety, Depression, and ADHD should be treated by appropriate medical professionals.

GENERAL TIPS FOR MENTAL HEALTH

Drink tea. Whether it's black, green, yellow, or white, tea has been proven to have great benefits. It can significantly help to alleviate stress, and even help your digestion. This is also a great way to reach your daily intake of water. If you believe that caffeine has a negative impact on your misophonia, try herbal, caffeine-free teas.

Do yoga, or some other form of stress management. Yoga, Pilate, and other activities are great for your mind and your body.

Find things you love. When you're doing things you love, the bad doesn't seem as bad. Even if there are triggers momentarily, you are much more likely to recover in an environment that makes you happy.

Be creative. Creativity is like a cheap drug. You can paint, do crafts, photography, design, and just about anything that lets your brain wander and find interesting ideas to incorporate into an artistic form.

Make goals and work toward them. When you're achieving life goals you will feel better about yourself. Especially when these goals are being met to spite your misophonia. It can be a small goal, such as a healthier lifestyle, or seeing your mother more, or a goal as large as starting your own business. The point is that working toward your goal will be good for your mind and can help improve your life.

Use noise masking. Noise masking is very important for eliminating audial triggers from an environment. Times like sleeping, being on a bus, or simply in day-to-day life can benefit from the addition of white noise. White, pink, and brown noise can be found in the form of noise apps for phones, videos on a computer, fans, and noise generators. Similarly, television or music may do the trick if you're merely trying to tune out trigger noises and cover them. There are also comforting sounds like ocean music and other "calming" sounds. White, pink, or brown noise may be more effective because it tends to block out our ability to hear these noises altogether, but music or television can be helpful by creating a positive mood. It really depends on what you're looking for. Regardless of the noise that you choose to go with, it is very useful to prevent hearing a trigger. Masking is most effective as a preventative measure but can help lessen the effects once already triggered. Avoiding trigger sounds altogether is the best outcome, but that's not always possible. Remember that masking will not take away the anger and discomfort that you are feeling toward a trigger, but it will help you to not hear more of the sound.

DISTRACTION

This can be highly beneficial when trapped with a trigger. When you're in a car, on a bus, in class, or somewhere that you can't immediately leave, it's important to train your mind to focus on something else. It will not alleviate the entire trigger, but it can take your reaction from a ten to a two if you're good at distracting yourself. You can distract yourself in many ways. Distraction is an important tool when you cannot get out of the situation. I have been known to put up my school bag as a barrier in class in order to avoid movements, and I am also known for wearing earplugs in class or playing games on my computer or chatting up a friend on my computer when I am trying to get away from the trigger environment mentally. A friend can help via text or a chat service, and you can really alter your mindset by making the time go by faster. This will not completely alleviate the trigger, but it may make it a lot easier to manage.

Misophonia Worksheet

COMMUNICATION EXERCISE

How would you explain misophonia to a person who has never heard of the disorder?

_____

_____

_____

_____

_____

_____

_____

_____

_____

_____

IS AVOIDANCE ADAPTIVE OR MALADAPTIVE?

Whether or not *avoidance* is a maladaptive coping mechanism is something that psychiatrists and psychologists debate. In the view of some authors, avoidance is a maladaptive behavior because it can hinder social events and learning engagement and thus should be remedied. This view is simplistic and does not account for the lack of habituation that is shown in persons with misophonia. When we think of misophonia through the lens of sensory regulation and the fight-flight-freeze response, it is only natural that a person with misophonia would want to *avoid* a trigger or leave the room when it happens. The easiest way to not be distressed is to not be in the presence of the stressor!

Whether or not *avoidance* is maladaptive or adaptive depends on numerous factors, and almost all of them are up to the individual and by extension their families. Social expectations are largely cultural and whether something like family dinner is something to be adapted to and coped with or something that can be avoided will be situational. For some, the distress at mealtimes is so great that even the cultural desire to eat dinner with one's family is not enough to overcome the urge to flee. It is important to not judge too harshly in these situations—even if it is yourself that you are judging.

There is a degree in which avoidance is a maladaptive coping mechanism, and that degree is whatever line the person with misophonia has drawn in the sand. For some, there are hard boundaries that cannot be crossed such as restaurants or movie theatres. For others, these lines are more nuanced and some days they can handle it and other days they cannot. This variance is to be expected when we consider self-regulation and remember that misophonia varies based on the physiological, cognitive, and emotional needs of a person, and not just on hard assumptions.

Of course, if a person with misophonia has become overly withdrawn, lonely, or is avoiding relationships with their friends and family altogether, then this is a maladaptive behavior. However, it is possible that it is not necessarily misophonia causing this behavior, but rather a lack of accommodations and safety in the relationship which helps the person with misophonia stay present. Unfortunately, some triggers cannot be covered (such as the sound of a person's voice), so this can become tricky in these scenarios.

The answer to the question this chapter sought to answer—"Is avoidance adaptive or maladaptive?"—is that it entirely depends on how often the person is avoiding, why they are avoiding, and whether or not it is leading to more distress for the individual who is doing the avoiding. While that answer might seem convoluted, it is also one that might change through negotiating accommodations and developing coping mechanisms.

Misophonia Worksheet

COMMUNICATION EXERCISE

Was there a time in the past where you could have explained misophonia and did not? Why?

_____

_____

_____

_____

_____

_____

_____

_____

_____

_____

WHY PEOPLE WITH MISOPHONIA DON'T LIKE HOLIDAYS

Misophonia during family events can be a catalyst for emotional turmoil. This is something that can be hard to understand if you do not have the disorder and have never experienced the fight-flight-freeze reaction that comes with sensory stimuli. For family members who don't understand the condition, this can seem like the person with misophonia is not enjoying family time, or as though they are not valuing the connections with their family. This is an unfortunate misconception, as persons with misophonia are just as likely to value family time and become lonely as people without misophonia.

For people with misophonia, legs shaking, jewelry clanking, chewing dinner, Christmas lights, and numerous other stimuli can cause a reaction that other people might never think about. As we stay in that room with this stimuli, our bodies become tense, our palms sweat, and our heart rate rises. Eventually, we may feel a physical sensation and pain, while the tension becomes both mentally and physically unbearable.

This feeling does not go away until we are away from the stimuli. This is why people with misophonia often leave early, flee, or try to spend time in another room alone—seemingly avoiding their family. People with misophonia might hide or take frequent naps if the gathering is in a place that permits. This is not a way to stay away from family, but rather the nervous system becoming so taxed and so unbearably overloaded, that the only option to avoid feeling sicker and in more pain is to flee. For some, this can translate to migraines or flu-like symptoms for days after the event. The cost of staying in the room with a trigger and "sucking it up" can be

THE MIRACLE QUESTION

If you woke up tomorrow and you no longer had misophonia, how would you react? What would you do?

_____

_____

_____

_____

_____

_____

_____

_____

_____

_____

_____

_____

_____

_____

_____

_____

_____

_____

high for individuals with misophonia and is something that is even harder to explain because without living it, it almost seems dramatic.

If a person with misophonia tells you something is triggering them, they do not mean it is "annoying" and they do not mean that they are simply "bothered". Instead, what this means is that this stimulus is overloading their nervous system and causing more pain each time it happens, eventually becoming so intense that the consequences of not leaving become more lasting as time goes on. Essentially, misophonia is a full-body experience that leaves us so tired, so exhausted, and so physically and mentally sore that we may try to avoid this experience altogether and become withdrawn. Please don't think that your family member who doesn't enjoy gatherings doesn't love you. This condition is very hard to manage, and holidays often bring more stress and more sensory stimuli than any other time of the year. For persons with misophonia, we are stepping outside of our safety and comfort in many ways, and for many of us we will not be able to calm down until we are able to get back to our routines. These routines have been developed out of necessity, as they are our general ways of adaptive coping with misophonia.

Misophonia Worksheet

COMMUNICATION EXERCISE

If the person you are explaining misophonia to does not believe
you, what would you say?

_____

_____

_____

_____

_____

_____

_____

_____

_____

_____

YOU CAN GO ANYWHERE WITH MISOPHONIA

In 2019, I did something with misophonia (and misokinesia) that I had convinced myself for five years wasn't possible. I took not one, not two, but four flights (two of which were connections, but still). Due to my sensory processing difficulties, I had been convinced that I was locked into a geographic area only reachable by car, and certainly not by bus, which I still won't use. I learned a valuable lesson from this trip: the things we're afraid of are often worse in our heads. My fear of traveling wasn't based on what *did* happen—it was thoroughly based on what *could* happen. As a teenager who was depressed and had heavy anxiety, I always wanted to go to the United States. I dreamt of New York—of flying away and seeing the world. Misophonia made me think that traveling wasn't possible...

As I flew from Canada to the United States, I made it through customs. I made it through waiting areas by avoiding them. I sat in corners. I ate sushi. I made friends with a girl who worked at the bank at the airport. The trip wasn't just *trigger-light*—it was fun.

On the plane I survived by wearing an eye-mask, having a neck pillow, and wearing earplugs with noise-cancelling headphones. The trip went by without a scratch. Once I got to the airport, I kept my headphones on and avoided areas with people sitting down (leg shaking is a huge trigger). Since airports are large, this was fairly easy.

The most liberating part of my journey was realizing that I could do it. Despite my misophonia which can be pretty bad, and despite all of the pain and suffering this disorder caused, I was able to fly to wherever I wanted. I can go wherever I want in the world—and I'll be okay. I am not trapped by this disorder.

It's important to remember that even though misophonia might feel impossible to live with, we do have choices. We can decide what matters to us and find ways to enjoy the world around us. Yes, we might have to use coping skills and we might have to avoid some situations, but that doesn't mean that we are unable to go where we want. It doesn't mean that we can't find ways to be happy. To see the world. To look outside of a plane window and almost cry for joy as you see New York from the plane for the first time.

MISOPHONIA AND DEPRESSION

While the research may not be sufficient to say definitively that misophonia causes depression, I believe that for many of us, depression has become a part of our lives. Isolation, sadness, and loss of interest in activities all go hand in hand with misophonia. It can be a hard disorder to live with, and some of us take from this a very bleak perspective. I do, however, think that there is hope. Coping skills and research can offer viable remedies for misophonia, but we should also consider our mental health. If you believe that misophonia has caused depression (or heightened feelings of depression you already had), then you should talk to a mental health professional. Even though counsellors cannot fix misophonia, these clinicians are trained to help you manage your depression and help you live a fulfilling life.

I first started battling depression before I had even heard of the word *misophonia*. I have been fighting that fight since I was 13 years old, and I've learned a few things along the way. I've learned that there is a degree of grief and loss that comes with depression. You must accept the depression and learn to move on from it. A huge part of this process is asking for help and allowing professionals and those that love you to be welcome in your life. This can be a hard step but it's important. Misophonia may not be the complete *cause* of depression, but it can certainly contribute to the illness. The following is advice that I wish somebody had told me when I first learned I had depression at 13 years old:

- It's absolutely okay to not be okay.
- You can get through this.
- Even though today is horrible it doesn't mean that tomorrow will be too.
- People want to help you. Be honest.
- Being depressed doesn't make you weird. It makes you human.
- If somebody doesn't believe you're depressed, then that's their problem. Your feelings are legitimate.
- There's no magic pill, but that doesn't mean you shouldn't try and help yourself.
- Some days are better than others.
- There's nothing wrong with staying in bed.
- There's nothing shameful in crying.
- Try to do something you love every day, even if you're not interested anymore. You'll be surprised when the good moments "peer through the curtain".
- Go outside. Even if you have to wear headphones. Breathe in fresh air.
- Take care of yourself. Take a shower. Eat.

- If you are clinically depressed, or suicidal, please call a hotline or immediately tell a relative, call 911, or go to an ER! Your life is important. You matter.

For the most part, I had recovered from depression when I discovered I had misophonia in 2014. I had good days, and I had bad, but my life was starting to get back on track. My life was finally starting to come together, and in my *Thought Catalog* article I explained that this was like crawling out of one hole to trip into another. As you can imagine, misophonia now triggers my depression at times. Even as I have become secure in other aspects of my life, and finally carved my own path, misophonia still leads to some of my darker moments. Misophonia is *hard*.

It is unfair and hard to live with the realization that some of your social relationships are fractured and may never fully recover because of the bitter pill that is misophonia. Living day to day in fear of triggers, feeling trapped and isolated, is even harder.

There may not be a cure for misophonia, but the sense of loss, hopelessness, anxiety, and depression that go along with it are treatable. Try to separate these things and treat the symptoms of depression. In doing so, you might become more equipped for handling triggers and the depression that follows. It's not a blanket cure, but you might be able to find good in the moments where no triggers are present. Do remember that research is happening. We're not alone. Even if it feels that way. It's going to be okay.

Misophonia Worksheet

REFRAMING MISOPHONIA

Example

Misophonia thought: Why did he have to whistle? It is so rude. I hate whistling. This is so cruel.

Misophonia thought re-framed: He probably does not know that whistling upsets me. Maybe he is happy or trying to keep himself calm.

Misophonia thought:

_____

_____

_____

_____

_____

_____

_____

_____

Misophonia thought re-framed:

_____

_____

_____

_____

_____

_____

_____

_____

IT'S OKAY TO GRIEVE

Misophonia is a life-altering condition with no existing treatment aside from coping skills; therefore, it is important that sufferers focus on what this means for them. It is important not to push these feelings away and feel guilty for having them. Grief must be dealt with and allowed to go through its stages. Once you grieve, you can accept that this is not the end of the world and that you can still make a life for yourself. Grieving is not about giving up, it is about letting go, and moving forward with the changes that have to be made. There are five stages of grief that were originally proposed in the book *On Death and Dying* in 1969 by Elisabeth Kübler-Ross. The stages of grief do not necessarily happen in order, and you can go from depression back to anger or any other combination. I should also mention that despite widespread proliferation, the stages of grief are not scientific in nature. These stages are meant as an explanation of grief and should not be applied rigidly. Nevertheless, these stages do offer a reasonable explanation for grieving.

THE 5 STAGES OF GRIEF

1. Denial and Isolation: Denial can come in different ways. People with misophonia may at first believe that they're just "hyper-sensitive" or that it's their fault. Isolation is huge for misophonia. A large number of sufferers spend most of their time alone and choose jobs and activities where triggers will not bother them. While this may help to prevent triggers, it is not a meaningful way to spend all of your time. Personal relationships and social interactions are a large part of happiness. Alone time is great, but it should not be all of your time.

2. Anger: It makes sense to be angry with misophonia. It's a life-changing, existence-altering condition. Even when you finally find out that you're not crazy and there's a name for it, you're faced with a harsh reality. There's currently no cure, and that's enough to make anybody angry. Of course, it's not fair that you have to suffer from this and that you can't just be "normal." However, the fact is that you have it and you're going to have to move on. Yes, your anger is warranted. However, you can't risk the rest of your life and your happiness because of this condition.

3. Bargaining: Sufferers may try to find help in ways that have a small chance of working. This can involve using therapies that have either not been tested or approved or have little evidence to support that they will work. While these methods can be very helpful for personal acceptance, it is not helpful if done out of desperation. Lack of results may put you further down a path of anxiety and depression and heed your progress.

4. Depression: It is easy to get depressed when things seem so bleak. Misophonia has been known to cause depression so severe that hopelessness and thoughts of suicide are possible. If this happens to you, then you should contact a mental health professional. It is important that you are properly equipped with coping mechanisms to help you through these emotions. Depression from grief is normal, but if it becomes too intense and endangers your life, then medical attention is a necessity. Do not feel guilty or be afraid that you might be judged if you need to ask for help. It shows great strength to seek the help that you need. Whether through therapy or soul searching, you must process your negative emotions and come to terms with them.

5. Acceptance: Misophonia may be a chronic condition but that does not mean that you will not be able to live a meaningful life. Once you accept misophonia, it will be easier to focus on coping methods and creating the kind of life that you want to live.

Misophonia Worksheet

EXAMINING THE MISOPHONIC MOMENT

What is the trigger?

_____

_____

Who or what is the trigger emanating from?

_____

_____

Why is the trigger sound/visual being made?

_____

_____

Is there anything adaptive you can do to stop it?

_____

_____

How can you adapt to the trigger if it cannot be stopped?

_____

_____

LONELINESS AND MISOPHONIA

Misophonia is an isolating disorder. Even as a married woman, I still feel the loneliness that accompanies this disorder. This loneliness can encompass many parts of one's life. The inability to engage in social activities as much as we would like, even including weddings and funerals, can be horrible to deal with.

I wrote the following piece after the death of a loved one, posted on *The Mighty* in 2017:

I have lost a lot from my disorder. Misophonia causes a fight/flight/freeze response to visual and audial stimuli. Whistling, chewing, leg-tapping, and other normal events become noxious to me. It is painful. There is no "ignoring" this. Once my amygdala faces a trigger, there is only escape. If I do not escape, the pain builds. Since this is accumulative, if I do not escape, I can end up with a migraine. I can get sick.

This week, I have lost something much greater, much sharper, much harder to deal with. A woman I love dearly, and will with every breath that goes forward, passed away. I come from a Catholic family, and grieving is something not only expected but enshrined in community.

News surrounding misophonia mostly focuses on "chewing rage," on the family impact, or on the inability to comply with day-to-day life-events. Misophonia, in this outreach, has gone beyond that. It has taken away my humanity, my ability to say goodbye to someone I love.

Unlike many I have talked to, I have not had misophonia my entire life. Some consider this lucky. I do not wish to discuss the implications of childhood vs. late-onset. That is not part of this story. The story is that I have buried many loved ones. I have been present at funerals, wakes, and have taken part in the grieving process. I know these events do not "solve" death. What I have learned from wakes and funerals is that to move on from death, and the loss of a loved one, we must be together.

As an advocate I have talked about misophonia's impact on my life time and time again. I feel as though I have a deep and meaningful relationship with coping with this disorder. I feel failed by all of this. I feel lost, sad, and scared. More, I feel as though I have had an important spiritual and life event stolen away from me.

I must move forward on a path of grieving that redefines my views. I am trying to move forward and respect the life of a loved one without being able to fully engage with her loved ones. I am trying to move forward, alone, in a way that respects my love for her. I don't know how to do this. I do not know how to sit alone in a room and quietly show loud respect for a woman who I believe deserves better from me. I wish I could have sat there in the room. I wish I could have shared in the grief of family, friends, and other loved ones. I could not.

I am grieving her loss. I am grieving my loss of grieving. I feel guilty for not grieving "properly." I feel guiltier still, that my own problems have overshadowed my grief for her. I know there are no answers. I feel lost, and I feel sad.

This is not necessarily a story of hope; it is a story of loss. Loss of self. Loss of love. It is a story of finding meaning in a silent room. I know her love surrounds me, but I do not know how to share this without being able to face a crowd. What I do know is disorders are important. I know it is important to show love and kindness to others, especially those in pain. I know this because people like her have taught me. As a nurse, Anne-Marie showed me kindness and compassion have the power not only to change the world around you, but the whole world.

Disorders like misophonia require constant advocacy. The world does not know us. We are not merely patients; we are people *in pain. We are humans who are loving, losing, and finding new ways to find love for each other.*

As advocates and as people, we must ensure the world we are creating is one that has more love for others. We must realize that even when we do not have the answers, we are capable of caring for each other. Even in our struggles, we must understand that if not for people and if not for love, what are we fighting for? While I may not be able to mourn in a room full of others, I can profess my love to the world. I can tell the universe that she was here. I can tell the world that her love now lives in all she's touched and will continue to grow and change the world.

Loneliness can manifest in many ways. My above example shows how misophonia can have deep cultural implications for a person, and even religious and spiritual fallout. With that said, I now try to attend events even if there are triggers. While I know this is uncomfortable, I have decided that the guilt associated with missing these events haunted me more than the potential stimuli. Neither choice is right or wrong, and it is up to each individual to decide what they value.

THE SENSORY DIET
Sensory Diet for Teenagers and Adults
By Susan Nesbit, M.S., OT.

Patricia and Julia Wilbarger coined the term *sensory diet*. Persons with sensory over-responsivity (SOR)—a subtype of sensory processing disorder (SPD)—use sensory diets to stay calm, energized, and organized. Sensory diets are used for SOR in many sensory channels, including the auditory (sounds), the visual (sights), the tactile (touch), and the olfactory (smells). The term SPD often is used interchangeably with SOR, including *auditory over-responsivity*. To be in sync with others, I use the term SPD in this document, unless the narrower term of SOR or auditory responsivity is needed for clarity.

Whether a sensory diet is also helpful for persons with misophonia is unclear. Sensory diets were developed to treat SOR. If the causes of misophonia are different, then a sensory diet may not be effective. Scholars have speculated that both conditions are neurologically based, and perhaps the same structures in the brain are involved. Scholars have additionally proposed that the limbic system plays a role. The limbic system controls our emotions and the fight-flight-freeze response. The amygdala filters out unimportant and irrelevant sensory information so that it does not reach the limbic system. Deep pressure and slow movement are theorized to help the amygdala act as a filter. If the amygdala plays a role in misophonia, then a sensory diet could lessen the impact of the triggers so that people can respond with less adversity to noxious sounds (triggers). Research is needed to investigate the similarities and the differences between auditory over-responsivity and misophonia.

The purpose of a Sensory Diet is to use a strategic mix of sensory activities to reduce *meltdowns* (e.g., yelling or snapping at someone) and *shutdowns* (withdrawing). Similar to eating food every few hours, the body must be replenished with sensory input. You may need to do a sensory diet every one to two hours. Sensory diets can be used at specific daily time periods or as needed. Choose one or more activities. Doing a sensory diet for 5-15 minutes can be helpful; however, doing a sensory diet for 30 minutes has a longer-lasting effect.

Proprioceptive (pressure) and vestibular (movement) inputs can be calming and organizing. Swinging is the ideal source of *vestibular* input. The effect in the brain from 15 minutes of swinging is reported to last up to eight hours.

Other types of sensory input affect the brain for one to two hours. Some experts recommend swinging for at least 15 minutes, two times per day (e.g., early morning and late afternoon). Because a swing hung from one hook can be moved at varying speeds (e.g., fast) and in more directions, using a swing hung from a single hook gives more intense and longer-lasting input than a swing hung from two hooks. Important points: slow, linear, and rhythmical movements are calming, and fast, rotary, and erratic movements are excitatory.

Proprioceptive input is speculated to help integrate vestibular input. Climb and jump after swinging. Proprioceptive input can be used alone without vestibular input. Proprioceptive input is obtained through "heavy work" such as carrying books, moving furniture, vacuuming, and lifting free weights. Proprioceptive input can be calming, energizing, and organizing, so when in doubt, use heavy work (proprioception).

NOTES ON OTHER TYPES OF SENSORY INPUT

Auditory (sounds): Many persons with auditory over-responsivity or misophonia can avoid becoming overwhelmed by controlling and predicting the noxious sounds (triggers), so take some control over environmental noises whenever possible.

Visual (sights): Visual input can be over-arousing for persons with auditory sensitivities. Simplify your visual field for a calming and organizing effect. Avoid clothes, towels, rugs, wall colors, etc., in colors that you find distressing. In contrast, if you feel "tuned out", add brightly colored objects to encourage visual attention.

Tactile (touch): Tactile input can be over-arousing. Light touch can be noxious; firm touch can be calming. Avoid clothes with labels, etc., that you find distressing.

Olfactory (smells): Odors calm, stimulate, or send a person into sensory overload. Persons with olfactory over-responsivity can become upset by something "stinky."

PRECAUTIONS

Avoid using lavender products with boys who have not yet reached puberty. In several recent studies, researchers found a link with breast growth. Experts also suggest not using these products with girls because the effects are not yet known. Lavender also has precautions for adults. When applied to the skin, for example, it sometimes causes irritation.

Other oils can cause irritation when applied directly to the skin. Experiment on small patches of skin before applying oils in large quantities. Putting a few drops into a warm bath can lower the risk of skin irritation. You can use a diffuser to dispense the oils; however, this method has a less intense impact.

Women who are pregnant or breastfeeding should avoid some of the oils listed below. Some of them should be discontinued two weeks prior to surgery, as they can negatively interact with the anesthesia. If you have pets in the home, please be mindful of what essential oils you diffuse as some are poisonous to animals. You should also never diffuse in a room from which a pet cannot escape.

CHOOSING YOUR SCENTS

Explore the scents to find the ones that best meet your needs, whether this is calming or alerting, and to find the aromas that you prefer. Scents that generally are calming and relaxing are lavender, rose, rosemary, chamomile, ylang-ylang, vanilla, and frankincense. Scents that generally are alerting without causing over-stimulation include citrus extracts which are the best oils for feeling awake (e.g., bergamot, grapefruit, orange, lemon, and lime), mint (e.g., peppermint and spearmint), pine (e.g., juniper and white fur), eucalyptus, and some herbs and spices (e.g., basil, rosemary, and cinnamon).

GUIDELINES

For people with SPD, the activities listed in this sensory diet are suggestions. The ideas are not intended to be cookbook recipes. Consider buying the book for the Alert Program to identify your level of arousal and the activities that are calming, energizing, and organizing for you. Alternatively, consult with an occupational therapist for a thorough evaluation and an individualized sensory diet. Use activities based on your interests. Start with something simple and gradually move on to something more challenging. Routines can be important. However, occasionally changing the routine might help you expand your interests if you desire to do so.

Pay attention to your mind/body. Notice when you need to cool off or calm down. Watch for signs that you are starting to relax after switching to calming activities. Activities that work for you one day may not work for you on a different day. Although a sensory diet has consistencies, variations occur from day to day and moment to moment, based on the noxious stimuli that have accumulated on that day at that moment.

Although I listed a particular activity once, putting it into only one category—calming, energizing, or organizing— some of the activities can be used in more than one category. Heavy work (defined as pushing and pulling against resistance and carrying heavy items) can be calming, energizing, and/or organizing. Use a strategic mix of sensory activities by paying attention to your mind/body. When in doubt, use heavy work (proprioception).

Borrowing the wisdom from the quote, "If you know one person with autism, then you know one person with autism", one can say, "If you know one person with SPD, then you know one person with SPD." In other words, all persons with SPD are unique individuals. As a result, the sensory diet that works for one person might not work for another person. Talk with an occupational therapist regularly, when possible, to be certain the sensory diet continues to fit your sensory needs.

Sensory diets should include calming, energizing (alerting), and organizing activities to be used based on your performance. Develop an individualized sensory diet using the lists below as a guide. Use calming activities during periods of high arousal or stress and energizing activities during periods of low arousal or calm.

CALMING ACTIVITIES

If you are over-stimulated, the following activities may help to calm you.

- Hugging/bear hugging with a partner.
- Tightly wrapping your arms around your torso and/or crossing your legs and/or squeezing your hands together.
- Cuddling with a partner or pets.
- Getting a firm massage or backrub with deep/firm pressure—light touch or stroking could be alerting.
- Pushing against a wall with back, buttocks, hands, head, or shoulders.
- Pushing against a wall as if to move it.
- Leaning forward with hands on edge of desk or table— gently pushing as if to move it; doing pushups if table is stable.
- Pushing into a chair with hands on the sides; holding self above chair with both arms; doing chair pushups.
- Rolling up tightly in a blanket.
- Slow rocking in a sleeping bag.

- Slow rocking, e.g., in a rocking chair.
- Swinging with slow, linear, and rhythmical movements (e.g., on a hammock).
- Carrying books or other heavy objects across a room or up and down the stairs.
- Wearing a heavy backpack (precautions: the cautious estimate to prevent injuries is to carry no more than 10% of your body weight, with 15-20% being less cautious estimates; use a backpack with wide and padded shoulder straps, a padded back, and a waist strap; distribute the load so it does not become bottom-heavy or top-heavy, and wear the backpack across both shoulders).
- Wearing a heavy backpack while carrying a few books.
- Wearing weighted collars, pillows, or blankets (heed precautions, especially with weighted vests).
- Taking a slow walk at sunset.
- Walking/strolling in a park.
- Swimming laps.
- Lifting free weights.
- Carrying a laundry basket.
- Washing windows, mirrors, or tables.
- Pushing and pulling heavy items (e.g., yard work)— mowing the lawn (with a push lawn mower), raking,

shoveling dirt or snow (heed safety precautions to avoid straining), and pushing firewood in a wheelbarrow.

- Enjoying leisure activities (e.g., reading or listening to books on tape) in a quiet space filled with pillows for cuddling (avoid over-stimulating visual distractions—use dim lighting, close the drapes/shades or sit with your back to the windows, use solid-colored furniture and rugs versus patterned ones and solid-colored walls in soft or neutral colors versus patterned wallpaper in bold colors, hide clutter in bins or boxes or behind doors or curtains— e.g., hang a solid-color curtain over a bookshelf, avoid wearing clothing in colors that you find distressing, and consider asking your loved ones, friends, and colleagues to avoid wearing clothes in colors that you find distressing).
- Watching fish swimming in an aquarium.
- Watching and listening to flames in a bonfire or fireplace, especially a fireplace with real wood.
- Listening to rain, waterfalls, and ocean waves.
- Listening to a tabletop fountain or an aquarium.
- Listening to quiet/soothing/relaxing classical music such as Mozart, Bach, Handel, Pachelbel, and Vivaldi.
- Listening to colored noise (e.g., white, pink, and grey); however, some persons find colored noise to be irritating.

- Taking a warm bath or shower before rolling up in a large towel (avoid using towels in colors that you find distressing).
- Using calming scents such as lavender and/or rose in oils, soaps, lotions, or candles (strong scents can be alerting rather than calming, so experiment).
- Wearing compression clothing, e.g., short-sleeved and long-sleeved t-shirts, shorts, and pants.

ENERGIZING ACTIVITIES

If you need to be aroused, wake up your senses by trying some of these activities:

- Tug-of-War (pull on a TheraBand tied around the doorknob of a closed door; use the strongest resistance possible).
- Pulling heavy items, e.g., suitcase or backpack on wheels.
- Jumping jacks/star jumps on the floor.
- Jumping on a mini trampoline (use a backyard trampoline if one is available).
- Jumping rope.
- Bouncing on a hopper ball, exercise ball, or therapy ball (these balls come in adult sizes).
- Brisk/vigorous walking and race walking.
- Hiking uphill.

- Stair climbing—race up the stairs, then go up the stairs two at a time (to cool off, walk at a normal pace down the stairs).
- Aerobics, including chair aerobics.
- Calisthenics, e.g., lunges, squat jumps, sit-ups, pushups, and pullups.
- Tumbling, e.g., cartwheels.
- Swimming—doing flips and somersaults in the water.
- Swing dancing.
- Spinning in rotating chair or on swing suspended from one hook.
- Using playground swings or a merry-go-round (you are never too old!).
- Taking a cool shower.
- Using alerting scents such as citrus, mint, and/or pine in oils, soaps, lotions, or candles.

ORGANIZING ACTIVITIES

These activities may calm or energize, depending on your needs. Pay attention to your body for signs that indicate your level of arousal.

- Squeezing stress balls.
- Sucking, e.g., water from a squeeze bottle, a popsicle, or a lifesaver.

- Sucking drinkable (liquid) yogurt through a straw.
- Eating healthy crunchy foods like carrots or chewy foods like jellybeans.
- Chewing bubblegum.
- Blowing soap bubbles.
- Climbing stairs (up and down) or a ladder.
- Doing pushups (on the floor from knees or toes; standing and leaning forward against a wall).
- Doing situps.
- Doing jumping jacks.
- Tumbling and gymnastics.
- Doing headstands or handstands against a wall.
- Hiking, walking, or running.
- Roller skating, roller blading, or ice skating.
- Jumping rope.
- Biking/cycling.
- Horseback riding.
- Stretching, including tai chi and yoga.
- Lying on your stomach to read a book.
- Painting the walls with plain and/or textured paints, e.g., add sand to the paint.
- Pushing heavy items, e.g., shopping cart, laundry basket, or box filled with books.

- Pulling heavy items, e.g., wagon filled with children, books, or laundry detergent.
- Vacuuming—especially when pushing the furniture out of the way!
- Taking out the rubbish/garbage/trash or hauling bags of leaves to the curb.
- Creating a scrapbook—ripping/tearing paper, using different textures, gluing (squeeze bottle) or pasting, and painting.
- Coloring mandalas—begin at the center and work your way to the outside border; use colored pencils or crayons because markers leak and destroy the experience.
- Sewing, knitting, crocheting, and weaving.
- Sculpting—making things out of clay through coil or slab methods; try using a potter's wheel.
- Woodworking—sawing, gluing in dowels, pounding nails, screwing in nuts and bolts, using sandpaper to smooth the project.
- Baking—mixing the ingredients in a bowl (not using an electric mixer) and squeezing/kneading, flattening, and rolling the dough for bread or cookies.
- Cooking—pounding chicken cutlets with a food hammer and chopping vegetables.

- Gardening—digging, patting soil, pulling weeds, carrying and pouring water from a large watering can, and pouring/dumping dirt or mulch.

ORGANIZING GAMES AND PARTNERSHIP OR GROUP ACTIVITIES

- Tug-of-War.
- Tennis or badminton.
- Softball or baseball.
- Volleyball.
- Basketball.
- Kickball or soccer.
- Martial arts, including taekwondo and karate.
- Races, e.g., adult relay races, 5K and 10K runs, half and full marathons, and track and field.
- Dancing and singing.

EXAMPLE OF A SENSORY DIET

Personalize this example. To meet your changing sensory needs, modify the activities as your needs change. Use a strategic mix of activities.

General suggestions: Take frequent movement breaks, sit on an inflatable wobble cushion, and chew crunchy foods (e.g., carrots) during daily activities that require attention and concentration. Rocking gently before bedtime can help with a sleeping problem. Try a firm self-hug after rocking.

IN THE MORNING:

- Upon awakening, massage your neck and shoulders— gently but firmly move your fingers in small circles—start at the base of your skull and move down your neck and then out toward one shoulder and repeat toward the other shoulder—work out the knots—then stretch by hugging yourself.
- Take a bath or a cool shower with alerting scents such as citrus, mint, or pine.
- Use a vibrating toothbrush and/or a vibrating hairbrush.
- Listen to music that you find alerting but not over-stimulating.
- Eat crunchy cereal with fruit and some protein.

- Take a brisk or vigorous walk or jump on a mini trampoline.

MIDAFTERNOON:

- Do aerobic exercises or jump on a mini trampoline.
- Go for a bicycle ride or do yoga.
- Push a grocery cart or a stroller, depending on family needs.
- Massage your feet to "reorganize".
- Listen to music that you find alerting but not over-stimulating.
- Oral work—suck liquid yogurt through a straw, eat crunchy and chewy snacks, or chew gum before and/or during activities at a desk or table.

AT DINNERTIME:

- Make a meal involving mixing, chopping, pounding, and so on.
- Set the table using two hands to carry and balance a heavy but stable tray.
- Eat crunchy and chewy foods.

AT NIGHT:

- Take a walk/stroll in a park.
- Sew, sculpt clay, or make woodworking projects or scrapbooks.
- Color mandalas—begin at the center and work your way to the outside border; use colored pencils or crayons.
- Take a warm bath with bubbles and calming essential oils such as lavender or rose.
- Give yourself a massage.
- Listen to quiet/soothing/relaxing music. This can be any music that you personally enjoy.

Misophonia Worksheet

PLANNING YOUR SENSORY SPACE

Where is your sensory space?

_____

_____

_____

_____

What items do you already have that you can add to your
sensory space?

_____

_____

_____

_____

What changes could you make to your sensory space to
make it calmer?

_____

_____

_____

_____

When will you come to your sensory space?

_____

_____

_____

_____

COPING SKILLS YOU CAN EASILY INCORPORATE

Passive coping skills are coping skills that you can incorporate into your life with little to no additional effort. Active coping skills require a little more planning, so they should be chosen carefully. The goal is to choose activities that fit into your life and that do not overwhelm you.

Passive Coping Skills	Active Coping Skills
Sleeping with a weighted blanket.	Sew, sculpt clay, do woodworking projects, or scrapbook.
Shower or bath steamers/bombs for scent therapy.	Make a meal involving mixing, chopping, pounding, and so on.
An essential oil diffuser in your room.	Carrying books or other heavy objects across a room or up and down the stairs.
Changing your curtains to a light-blocking style.	Swimming laps.
Wearing a heavy weighted vest.	Switching to taking stairs instead of an elevator.
Listening to colored noise (e.g., white, pink, and grey).	Going for regular walks, and even better if they are in a calming nature environment.

Fill out your own passive/active coping skills list.

Passive Coping Skills	Active Coping Skills

HOW MISOPHONIA IMPACTS RELATIONSHIPS

Since misophonia isn't a widely known disorder, it is important that those who suffer are well equipped to explain their condition to parties who could be causing a trigger or to those who are able to provide support for misophonia. Persons with misophonia should realize that the nature of the relationship will change how you explain the condition, or how you might respond in the event of triggers emotionally.

Regardless of who it is you are explaining misophonia to, be assertive when you state that you have the disorder. You can be polite and assertive at the same time. Explain that misophonia does not mean that you are making excuses for yourself, it merely means that you are explaining your disorder. If a person does not understand but shows interest, offer to send them links to sites on misophonia. Tell them that it's reasonable that they don't know, but that there is growing research on the disorder. Before arranging to meet with a new person, I briefly explain my disorder. I explain that certain sights and sounds give me a fight or flight reaction and ask that they keep them to a minimum. I have had much more success explaining this before a meeting than in the moment when being triggered, which is essentially too late. Different relationships have different considerations, and I have listed some of these variabilities below—however, this is not a catch-all, merely a suggestion of some possible scenarios.

EXPLAINING MISOPHONIA TO PEOPLE YOU SEE OFTEN

This section has reminders for the steps to take when explaining misophonia to your boss, friends/co-workers, family, and other persons who are in your life on a regular basis.

- Only explain misophonia for the first time when you are not triggered if possible.
- Bring the results of a misophonia assessment and/or accommodations list in letter form to the conversation (most helpful for work but can also help for some doubtful families).
- Focus on the way the trigger makes you feel and the sound/visual, *not* the person making the sound/visual.
- Acknowledge that accommodating misophonia can be hard and express gratitude when you are accommodated.
- Provide resources such as the Printout Guides on the IMF website, links to scientific articles, and other explanations that are formalized.

FAMILY

Those nearest and dearest are often the worst triggers. We spend a lot of time with our loved ones and, in general, we seem less forgiving when it comes to their behaviors. Day in and day out with the same people can be stressful for anyone. Even if you do not live with a family member, the intensity of the relationship can still cause misophonia triggers to be worse. My first ever "trigger person" that I knew was my mother. At first, every time she shook her foot it was a major fight. We're talking volcanic eruption on both sides. You didn't want to be there when she played music and when she sang. I know it isn't her fault that she does these things, and they never used to bother me. Misophonia doesn't always make sense. Explaining misophonia to family members often involves a lot of conversations surrounding the disorder, offering resources, and reassuring family that it is not *them* that you are mad at, and that it is the disorder causing these negative emotions.

FRIENDS

I now refuse to spend time recreationally with people who do not respect my misophonia. It was a hard adjustment at first, but the people who truly care about me are able to respect misophonia. Friendship, like dating, should be based on a mutual understanding and trust. You should not have to pressure your friend to respect your needs and wishes. Be sure to explain to your friend that you do not mean anything by your displeasure, and that you truly value their time and your relationship. Ask if you can have gatherings in trigger-neutral zones and plan your outings so that the possibility of a trigger is minimal. This can be hard since a lot of friendships involve activities that involve noises or visual stimuli. Try to pick outings that have noises that you are comfortable with. For example, I am fine with the sound of bowling balls and pins crashing. Bowling is a great way for me to hang out with friends because most of the people I can see are standing, which means not shaking any body parts, and the rest of the facility is usually dark. A great friend will understand that you are not doing this to be nitpicky and will want to make you feel at ease. However, you must understand that they have emotions too, and that you should try not to attack them when triggered.

ROMANTIC PARTNERS

Misophonia is often the cause of distress in relationships where one of the members has misophonia. Your partner clinks their spoon in a bowl, taps their fingers, or shakes their legs. Maybe they like to whistle. At first, you may try to ignore it, but eventually the triggers can become worse and worse. The honeymoon phase is over, and misophonia changes all of your emotions. Like friends and family, you need to be able to discuss your misophonia with your partner. Hard work and honesty are going to be the key in going forward. Your partner must respect your condition and know the role it plays in your life, and you must understand and respect your partner's emotions when it comes to being the trigger and living their life with you.

ROOMMATES

Like family, these people are there on a day-to-day basis. However, unlike family, there may not be enough of a personal relationship that you can confront the individual in a positive manner. Sometimes, our living arrangements are out of our control. You may be living in a dorm room, an apartment, or another communal situation. Money and other uncontrollable forces often lead to the necessity of living with a stranger, or even an acquaintance. Ideally, we would never live with someone whom we didn't have a good relationship with. Unfortunately, reality isn't always a perfect picture. If you're going to be living with a new person, you should discuss your misophonia before moving in. Try to be sure that the person you're going to live with truly understands your needs and establish ground rules. Explain that you are not trying to dictate them and that you are merely suffering from a neurophysiological condition. If they, or a current roommate, do not respect these ground rules, then perhaps you should consider a different living arrangement if possible. Living with your triggers should only be a last resort. While you cannot avoid triggers in every aspect of your life, the home should be a neutral place where you can relax and have a sanctuary for the sake of your health and sanity.

BOSS OR ADMINISTRATION

Your boss should be a person that you trust and that you can approach with issues that involve your work performance and comfort in the workplace. For some people, their boss is intimidating and a person to which they would rather not disclose personal medical details. If you do decide to have this conversation, it is best to arrive prepared. You should explain that misophonia is a neurophysiological condition for which there is little information and no cure yet. Ask your boss if there is anything they can do to help and assure them that you are committed to the job and are asking for the betterment of not just yourself, but your performance. If your boss is unsupportive, you should be prepared with the laws reflecting accessibility in your region.

CO-WORKERS

Co-workers can be tricky. This is especially worrisome for those that work in an office environment. The cubicle environment is especially hellish for persons with misophonia. A lot of workplaces are starting to allow snacking on the job, and this causes a lot of triggers. Being polite can go a long way with other workers, no matter the situation. However, sometimes coworkers aren't willing to stop something that they believe is "their right." Approach the co-worker when you aren't triggered and inform them that you have a medical condition and ask them if they would be willing to help accommodate you. If they are not willing to help and further the situation, inform your boss. You should already have told your boss about your misophonia and discussed the possibility of accommodations in this scenario. You may be able to convince your boss to speak with your co-worker or find more suitable work arrangements.

DOCTORS (AND OTHER MEDICAL PROFESSIONALS)

When faced with a medical struggle, most of us decide to go to a doctor. The trouble with misophonia is that many doctors have never heard of it. Most doctors will automatically assume that it is psychological and will refer you to a psychiatrist or a psychologist, or personally recommend medication. This can be frustrating and possibly infuriating. Depending on where you live, it may cost a lot of money to be thrown through hoops without knowing if you'll ever find a cure. It's best to do your research on doctors that provide help for misophonia. However, you should still have a conversation with your doctor and let them know what is happening with you. As research grows, your doctor may become interested in the disorder and could eventually help others, and maybe even you.

TEACHERS AND PROFESSORS

Dealing with professors and teachers can be its own kind of hell. Thankfully, most schools these days (at least universities, colleges, and technical schools) have great accessibility programs. They're not perfect, but they're getting a lot better. The hardest part of this seems to be intimidation. The entire system seems set up to make professors and teachers seem larger than life, and that can be intimidating. If your school wants you to discuss your condition with your professor, you must approach them when you are in a good mood. You should never approach your professor on a day on which you are triggered. I have been lucky enough to only have positive interactions with my professors in regard to my misophonia, anxiety, and depression. Remember that most teachers and professors are there to help you. They are not the enemy and they usually want their students to succeed. All of your interactions should be polite, considerate, and professional. Speak to the professor with kindness but firmness.

HAVING THE MISOPHONIA TALK

When you know that you have to tell a person about your disorder, it can be stressful. Consider the tips below when you're going to confront somebody. You may want to adjust the conversation depending on whom you're talking to, but these tips should help you when thinking about how to act, what to do, and what to say. It's a good idea to make sure you're not triggered at the time of the conversation. During a trigger, your anger is heightened and you may perceive the person as a threat. It's important that you are prepared to explain misophonia in a positive manner. No one wants to feel attacked. Prepare yourself with research and website links that can be helpful to explain misophonia to the person you're about to approach. Make sure that they will understand that it is a real condition, and that you are serious.

Keep your mood stress-free and ensure that you are relaxed beforehand. Try to have a bath, some tea, or some light television or something you enjoy before you have the conversation. Whatever makes you feel better. If you are stressed or tired, the conversation may go poorly quickly. Choose a location in which you know there will be little to no triggers. Try to be somewhere that you and the other individual are both comfortable. If this is impossible, try to become familiar with the place beforehand (such as talking to the person in their office and asking if you can meet another day when you have more time or are more prepared).

DURING THE CONVERSATION

During the conversation, your aim should be to keep it positive and informative. You should provide examples of what triggers you, even if they are not the *same ones* that trigger you in the environment with the person. It is important that they understand it is not just when you are around this person and that this disorder impacts several aspects of your life. Do not make it all about them.

It may be helpful to print off articles that explain misophonia and what it is. If the person triggers you during the conversation, identify it but not in an aggressive manner. Excuse yourself and explain that what they are doing is one of the things that causes a reaction. Politely ask if they can stop or if there is a way they can adjust their behavior. Make sure they understand you are not blaming them. If possible, do not apologize for misophonia or make excuses. Use this opportunity to discuss a way that you can let them know you are being triggered without being offensive or turning to anger. If the conversation starts to go sour or the person does not understand—excuse yourself and try again later, perhaps armed with a different resource.

AFTER THE CONVERSATION

Chances are that after you explain misophonia to another person they will still trigger you. It can be hard for a person to recondition things that they are used to doing, and even harder to remember. Unlike you, this person does not deal with misophonia on a day-in-day-out basis, so it's unlikely that it's something they consider regularly. Do not blame them for this and do not hold it against them. Unless the person is trying to trigger you and disregards your feelings entirely, you should be mindful that they are probably not out to get you, and that it is merely a reaction from misophonia. Below are some useful tips:

- If you have to remind them that they are triggering you, be polite.
- Leave the room and if they ask why, explain that you are being triggered.
- Try to remain positive; do not engage when you are angry.

THE OTHER SIDE OF THE FENCE

Hearing a sufferer explain her condition and also how she changes her lifestyle for her son gave me some ideas. For once, I wasn't the person explaining that I had the disorder; I was merely the person listening to the story. To say the least, it was strange to be on the other side of the fence. This is the side where you don't exactly know what to say and you're at a loss for words. In this section, I want to shed some light on this position. Hopefully, I can also help people without the disorder to understand what they could say to get around their confusion. There's a good chance that the person who is triggering you does not want you to feel such a negative reaction from their behavior. Even worse, they may feel guilty or like they're being blamed for your thoughts and feelings and that can be troublesome to live with. The following are considerations to make about the feelings of people who are your triggers, and what it may be like to be them.

I haven't always had misophonia. I can still remember days past when I wasn't bothered by or triggered by any noises. A person who doesn't have sensory processing issues or misophonia probably won't notice the sights or sounds that you're noticing. In fact, they may be so oblivious that they don't even know if they're making noise or moving. When you have misophonia, it's nearly impossible to imagine that these noises or visuals can be completely unseen and unheard. However, when you're not living with it on a daily basis, it can be very hard to understand what the big deal is about. A person without misophonia may wonder why you're so upset and first think you're merely hypersensitive. It's not their fault that they think this way. Each person has trouble seeing outside of their own experiences, so it's hard to consider the viewpoint of a person with misophonia.

A person who is triggering a loved one or a close friend may feel a significant amount of guilt when trying to deal with misophonia and its impact. After all, they do not want to hurt you. And yet, one wrong move and they're being given the stink-eye, yet again. It's traumatic to always be griped at and "attacked" for making a noise you're used to or moving a part of your body. Unfortunately, the person who is triggered has little control of their emotions in the moment. However, that doesn't mean that the feelings of the person who the misophonic response is directed toward does not feel it too. People have trouble considering changing their habits or behaviors in order to ease the lifestyle of another. It's not because they're arrogant or selfish; it's because everybody is just trying to get by in their own way. A significant amount of the population hums, whistles, or shakes their legs or sways when they are uncomfortable or faced with anxiety. Unfortunately, these behaviors tend to send people with misophonia into a rage, and this reaction could further send the person causing the trigger into anxiety. Misophonia is uncomfortable for everybody involved. I've always said that the worst-case scenario is a person with ADHD living with a person with misokinesia/misophonia.

The lack of medical knowledge and research on misophonia is not only challenging, but also very confusing for people who do not have it. If you think it is hard living with the disorder, imagine watching it happen but not knowing what to do, or whether or not your actions could actually be making the disorder worse. This is especially challenging for parents that are trying to guide their children in the right direction. A lot of people will say that their kids cannot be coddled and that they should be forcing them to "toughen up." This can send a mixed message to parents. Since the pain associated with misophonia is severe, a parent's reaction will be to protect their child—but a lot of people will be urging them to force their child to "get over it".

Misophonia is an emotional struggle for everybody involved. There are no right answers, and the current amount of research and diagnosis is so small that it's hard to feel a sense of hope once you know that it's, in fact, a real diagnosis. However, this does not mean it is all gray skies. Open communication can be helpful for everybody. If you are being triggered, you should be able to communicate this positively or, if that is the only excuse available, leave the room. If you are not the person suffering, but rather the trigger, or a person involved with a misophonia sufferer, you should learn not to take their behavior personally.

Misophonia Worksheet

CREATE YOUR OWN SENSORY DIET

In the morning:

_____
_____
_____
_____
_____

Midafternoon:

_____
_____
_____
_____
_____

At dinnertime:

_____
_____
_____
_____
_____

At night:

_____
_____
_____
_____
_____

MISOPHONIA ACCOMMODATIONS

If you have read *Misophonia Matters*, then these suggestions will be familiar to you. I am repeating them yet again because I believe they are incredibly important for coping with misophonia. I want to add that accommodation for the disorder is really our best way forward since there is no current way to alleviate the symptoms of misophonia entirely. Accommodating as much as we can is a great way to lower the overall stress surrounding misophonia and increase bandwidth for moments where we must—or want to—be present.

Before we can discuss how to negotiate misophonia accommodations, we must establish what accommodations are specifically. Misophonia accommodations are of course dependent on the needs of the individuals and their triggers, but the following lists will serve as examples of accommodations in various scenarios. For the purpose of potential accommodations, I will include both visual and auditory triggers. Each accommodation is offered as a suggestion; their viability is up to the individual, the parents of a child with misophonia, and the clinician working with a person with misophonia.

FAMILY ACCOMMODATIONS

Family accommodations are often dependent on the environment and are quite nuanced. However, this list serves as an example of what those accommodations might be.

- Wearing noise-cancelling headphones.
- Wearing earplugs.
- Eating family dinners in separate areas.
- Family bonding activities that do not involve food (board games, nature walks, etc.).
- A place in the house where the person with misophonia can retreat.

SCHOOL ACCOMMODATIONS

School accommodations refer to accommodations for ages from kindergarten to college.

- Wearing noise-cancelling headphones.
- Wearing earplugs.
- The ability to leave class if overstimulated.
- Online schooling if misophonia is impeding learning.
- A smaller and less overwhelming class.
- No eating in class if possible.
- A set seat/desk in the area where the person is most comfortable.

WORK ACCOMMODATIONS

When negotiating with human resources departments and managers, people with misophonia might ask for some of the following accommodations. This is dependent on whether or not it is feasible in their position. Some people with misophonia are adaptive and choose lines of work based on their triggers. The following may be helpful.

- Wearing noise-cancelling headphones.
- Wearing earplugs.
- A private office or cubicle away from others.
- The ability to work from home.
- A job that allows for flexibility in hours.
- No eating in meetings.

PUBLIC ACCOMMODATIONS

Public accommodation is impossible in the same way as other accommodation. For example, for the most part we cannot dictate which stores play which music or have specialized shopping trips. Public accommodations are more individually driven by proactively finding ways to cope with misophonia. Here are some suggestions.

- Wearing noise-cancelling headphones.

- Wearing earplugs.
- In waiting room situations, having a family member or friend wait in the room for you and text when it is your turn.
- Using a delivery or online ordering service to limit time in shopping environments.

SUMMARY LIST OF POTENTIAL MISOPHONIA ACCOMMODATIONS

- Wearing noise-cancelling headphones or earplugs.
- Calmly asking the triggering person if they would accommodate misophonia.
- Eating family dinners in separate areas.
- Family bonding activities that do not involve food.
- A place in the house where the person with misophonia can retreat.
- The ability to leave class if overstimulated.
- Online schooling if misophonia is impeding learning.
- A smaller and less overwhelming class.
- No eating in class if possible.
- A set seat/desk in the area where the person is most comfortable.
- A private office or cubicle away from others.
- The ability to work from home.
- A job that allows for flexibility in hours.
- No eating in meetings.
- In waiting room situations, having a family member or friend wait in the room for you and text when it is your turn.
- Using a delivery or online ordering service to limit time in shopping environments.

NEGOTIATING BOUNDARIES

Unfortunately, there are often triggers that cannot be avoided by the person with misophonia. An example of this is somebody who clears their throat or snores (barring sleep apnea which should get checked out). Some sounds are necessary. More than that, some sounds (and visuals) are part of activities that are important to our partners. This chart is meant to help couples negotiate their "Never", "Sometimes", and "Adapting" triggers. Adapting sounds are ones that are necessary or unavoidable. The adapting portion comes in to help the couple negotiate ways for the misophonia sufferer to live in this environment where triggers are present. The following example is my own chart based on my own triggers, but each couple will have a chart tailored to their situations. These categories can change over time! For example, restaurants used to be in my "Never" category. This list should not be treated like scripture but rather used for couples to identify their needs and boundaries.

SAMPLE BOUNDARY NEGOTIATION CHART

Never	Sometimes	Adapting
Whistling. Finger tapping. Gum chewing. Leg shaking.	Popcorn during movies. Going to restaurants.	Sneezing. Coughing. Chewing. Sharp S sounds when talking.

BOUNDARY NEGOTIATION CHART

Never	Sometimes	Adapting

WHAT IF YOU FEEL GUILTY OR BITTER THAT YOU NEED ACCOMMODATIONS?

Some people with misophonia have expressed to me that they feel uncomfortable always using assistive technology or accommodations for misophonia. I think it is important to consider these thoughts of *guilt* or *shame* that we might feel by using these technologies such as earplugs, sensory tools, earphones, or noise generators. Perhaps as a child you were told that your misophonia was a "you problem" and you internalized that you should "just get over it", or maybe you worry that others seeing you wearing these devices will judge you and think there is something wrong with you. It is natural to worry about the way those in our environment feel about us, and perhaps ironically, this is also part of threat detection. The outsider of a group has less safety as they do not have the protection of the collective.

When it comes to accommodating misophonia, I personally believe that sufferers should feel empowered to use the tools that help them mitigate the disorder. For example, we would not accost a person who is deaf for using hearing aids, and we would never berate a person in need of a wheelchair. While misophonia is not yet as accepted by the wider public, I think sufferers should at the very least show the same grace to themselves as they would to a stranger or a loved one suffering with a more "accepted" condition.

Misophonia is a lifelong struggle and thus it is a marathon and not a sprint. The tools that we learn to adopt for misophonia should be utilized as needed, without shame. It is my hope that the sufferers of misophonia and clinicians reading this book see accommodation and advocacy as the cornerstone to managing and mitigating misophonia.

WHY IS MISOPHONIA TRIGGERED MORE BY PEOPLE YOU LOVE?

Since we spend more time with our friends and family, it should be no surprise that their noises (and visuals) become some of our worst triggers. It can still be baffling to come to terms with the fact that our own mothers, fathers, or friends are causing us distress. It's important to note that while people we are close to may be our worst triggers, this doesn't mean that it's because of anything they or you have done.

While research has yet to identify the exact reason why loved ones trigger us more than others, Dr. Jennifer Brout offers her idea of why this happens. Sensory information is cumulative. Because of this, each time we are triggered we become more overwhelmed, and then we may react more quickly to a person around us. We're also more likely to trust that a family member or friend will still love us if we overreact! Another reason loved ones may trigger us falls more along the lines of our brain makeup—our memories. The more a person triggers us, the more likely we are to associate them with the sounds. Unlike someone without misophonia, we do not "get used" to a sound or experience.

Instead, it becomes a neverending nightmare. If you're anxious or tense around a person, you may be more likely to store triggers in memory. If a person is a trigger, you should try to handle the situation as calmly as possible. It's best to leave explaining your disorder for when you're calm. Escalating the situation is unlikely to repair the damage, and the negativity can just make your disorder worse.

While we can't always avoid trigger sounds, it can sometimes be best to leave the situation when your nervous system gets triggered, as you can sometimes become calm by removing the situation for a brief period of time. Leaving the situation can be helpful to

MISOPHONIA JOURNAL MOMENT: WHEN WAS THE LAST TIME YOU WERE TRIGGERED, AND HOW DID YOU CALM YOURSELF DOWN?

I encourage you to use the space on the side of this page to reflect on how you calmed down the last time you were triggered.

_____

_____

_____

_____

_____

_____

_____

_____

_____

_____

_____

_____

_____

_____

_____

readjust your nervous system. This can be hard for many, but it is something that can be adapted to over time. As Dr. Brout says, "There is no formula for when to avoid or to approach sounds. There's no right or wrong. It might be comforting to know that avoidance and escape from aversive stimuli is normal, and in fact, it's a survival mechanism".

On some days, triggers may be worse than others. This can be confusing for persons with the disorder. On some days, we can handle some of the triggers surrounding us, and on other day the drop of a pin can bring us to a full-swung panic. Your physiological arousal is actually worse when you're anxious, already in a bad mood, sick, or simply tired. Sensory cumulation also means that new trigger situations are more likely. With this in mind, it's important that we consider our health before going into a situation. While you shouldn't keep yourself away from fun activities, you should not feel guilty about needing more "alone time".

CREATING A FAMILY GENOGRAM

Genograms are a tool often used in Bowenian Family Systems Theory (Ungvarsky, 2022), and they may be helpful for families learning about their family history as it relates to misophonia and relationships between family members. Genograms are a way for therapists working with families, or individual families on their own, to record cognitively relevant family associations over generations. Genograms take effort and can be emotionally difficult to process, yet this is due to their enormous power when it comes to putting down on paper the history of a family. The members of the family involved in creating a genogram do not necessarily have to be all of the family, but rather this can be a useful tool for parents or misophonic members of the family to understand important connections and history that might be making it harder to negotiate misophonia. For example, the above scenario of restless leg syndrome and misophonia could be charted via a genogram.

You can use an online template for a genogram or download Genopro as a free trial to make a genogram. However, there is no reason to buy software for this exercise, as you can also use a piece of paper (or Bristol board). If you are working with small children, you could decorate your genogram with photographs if you like. For the purpose of

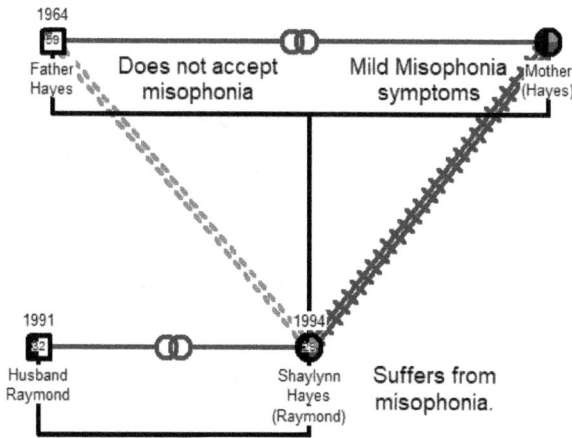

the example below, I sketched a conflict where my father does not accept misophonia. The red dotted bar indicates a conflict in a genogram.

The symbols for genograms can be confusing to learn at first, but it is important to remember that this is not a perfect exercise, but merely to help the family understand their dynamics. Important information to include in a genogram include family conflicts, genetic conditions (such as links

where multiple family members have misophonia), and
conditions that each family member has such as our example
of restless leg syndrome and misophonia. For a
comprehensive guide on genogram symbols, you can use the
in-depth guide from Edraw:
www.edrawsoft.com/genogram/genogram-symbols.html You
could also look into this software to help with your
genogram: https://www.wingeno.org/#windows

If you and your family choose to use a genogram, you
should remember that the exercise itself should not cause
conflict, but merely be used to highlight emotional and
genetic relationships that exist in the family. Bowenian
theory ascribes to the idea that if one family member makes a
change, the entire unit will be changed. Genograms are a tool
for understanding the family unit as a whole, and thus can be
helpful for identifying areas where negotiation or reflection
are necessary.

HOW TO ASK PEOPLE TO STOP TRIGGERING YOU WITHOUT BEING RUDE

As a person with misophonia, I am constantly uncomfortable and feel like the world is against me. I do not want to feel this way, but it is a fact that many of the sounds that trigger misophonia and the visuals that trigger misokinesia are ones that are made by other people or by machinery used by other people. Some of these include lawnmowers, loud bass music, rattling car engines and exhausts, and whistling, among others. I am not even mentioning chewing or sniffling because these are sounds that I genuinely think we cannot even bring up to strangers since they are necessary to life.

I have politely asked people in public to stop whistling. The way I explain this often goes like this:

Me: Excuse me, I am so sorry to ask, I have a hearing condition and I was wondering if you could please stop whistling? Again, I am so sorry to ask.

Yes, the Canadian in me says sorry twice. I hate inconveniencing people in general so asking them to change their actions to suit me is something I genuinely do not want to do. Yet, by asking politely, I have noticed that oftentimes people are happy to adjust. I will say that sometimes I feel far too aggravated and dysregulated to ask a person to stop, so the avoidance and resentment of my fellow humans starts to come into play.

I think the key to not being rude is to ensure that you are being polite and mindful of the other person, acknowledging that what they are doing is not wrong and that you are not entitled to their compliance, yet asking in a way that is kind and polite. If the person does not stop the behavior, unfortunately there is very little that can be done, so hopefully you do not have to be around them too often. If this is somebody you must be around every day (such as a colleague), then it would be reasonable to escalate the matter in my opinion, especially since (and only after) you tried to calmly and politely address the subject. This could be achieved by discussing options with your boss, consulting your human resources department, or asking your therapist to write you a note explaining misophonia.

SAMPLE ACCOMMODATION LETTER

Please note that this sample letter is provided as a sample only, so you must take this to your own practitioner if you'd like to use it. This note does not serve as its own accessibility note, and it is merely provided as a way to showcase what an accommodation letter might look like.

To Whom It May Concern,

My name is [Therapist Name] and I have been counselling [Client Name] for the past few months regarding a condition called misophonia, as well as for generalized anxiety and depression. While there is no official diagnosis for misophonia (nor could I diagnose as a counsellor even if there were), there is reliable and valid self-assessment from Duke University which I conducted via telehealth therapy with [Client Name]. On the Duke Misophonia Questionnaire, [Client Name] scored in the [range here] misophonia range, which indicates that symptoms of misophonia are causing a great deal of distress for [Client Name].

I am asking the receiver of this letter if you would consider accommodations for [Client Name] including:

- The ability to take their meals out and not be present in the lunchroom.
- A quiet place to wait or the ability to have another pickup location for their meal.
- I am available if you require further explanation regarding this accommodation.

Thank you for your consideration.
Sincerely,
Therapist Name

DECISION FLOWCHART

Some activities are important to our partners, and thus we should make an effort to take their interests, hobbies, and passions into account. Unfortunately, there are some activities which might not be possible for an individual with misophonia. Whether this activity can be substituted for another, done with modifications, or the partner can do the activity on their own or with a friend is entirely up to the couple. This flowchart aims to help you with these decisions. In the case that an alternative activity is chosen, the individual who is giving up their activity should be given first choice of a new more misophonia-friendly activity.

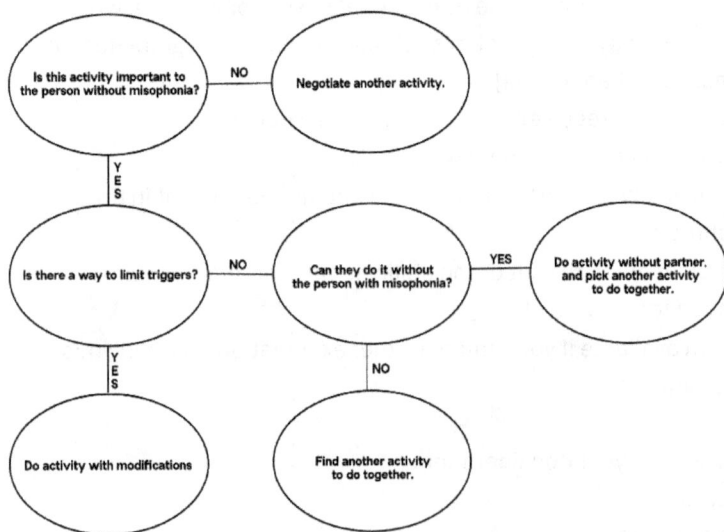

Is this activity important to the person without misophonia? — NO → Negotiate another activity.

YES ↓

Is there a way to limit triggers? — NO → Can they do it without the person with misophonia? — YES → Do activity without partner, and pick another activity to do together.

YES ↓ (Is there a way to limit triggers?) → Do activity with modifications

NO ↓ (Can they do it without the person with misophonia?) → Find another activity to do together.

ONLINE COLLEGES AND UNIVERSITIES

Going to school, especially university, is hard even without a disability. Misophonia further complicates matters. That's why I decided to switch from my brick and mortar school to an entirely online degree program. I want people to know that it is *not* a failure to go to an online school. In today's day and age, the resources have become exponentially better, and you'll often end up paying less, and having more time to get your studies completed. There may be more schools available than listed as this changes regularly; I highly suggest you do your own research if this is an avenue you'd like to explore.

IN THE UNITED STATES

CAPELLA UNIVERSITY

Capella offers a wide variety of programs from the Bachelor's to the PhD level. This is a very wide breadth of programs in a wide variety of topics and disciplines.

COLORADO STATE UNIVERSITY

From their website, "At CSU-Global, your online college tuition rate is what you pay. There are no additional student fees at any point in your academic journey. No out-of-state fees, no athletic fees, no per-credit fees, no additional fees period."

PENN STATE WORLD CAMPUS

From their site, "Penn State World Campus is ranked in the Top 10 for its online undergraduate and graduate programs among the hundreds of higher education institutions included in U.S. News & World Report."

MARYVILLE UNIVERSITY

Maryville offers 15 bachelor's degrees that fit seamlessly into your busy schedule. They all feature a flexible format, helpful transfer tips, and personalized support to help you succeed every step of the way.

IN CANADA

ATHABASCA UNIVERSITY

Athabasca University (also where I finished my BA) is a great option for Canadian students that want to obtain an entire BA over the internet. I switched here from brick and mortar and it's been a positive experience. A bonus is that the cost of your books and course materials is included in the price with no hidden fees. You can even take your exams online via Proctor U.

YORKVILLE UNIVERSITY

Like Athabasca, Yorkville is where I completed part of my studies. I attended Yorkville for their Master's program but the school also offers Bachelor's programs.

IN THE UK

THE OPEN UNIVERSITY UK

The Open University is the world's leading provider of flexible, high quality online degrees and distance learning or what is sometimes referred to as e-learning; serving students across the globe with highly respected degree qualifications, and the triple accredited MBA.

Misophonia Worksheet

REIMAGINING MISOPHONIA

Think of a time when you experienced a distressing situation involving misophonia. Perhaps this was in public, at school, or with a loved one. Instead of recreating this event, re-write the event in a way that you wish it had happened. You could include sensory-based strategies, psychoeducation (teaching the person about misophonia), or negotiating accommodations. How you re-write the scenario is up to you.

Your Reimagined Scenario

_____
_____
_____
_____
_____
_____
_____
_____
_____
_____
_____
_____
_____
_____
_____
_____
_____
_____

MISOPHONIA IN THE MEDIA

For a decade, I have been fighting the media like swatting flies with a fly swatter when it comes to misophonia and how it's represented in the media. This is a headache I will probably still be dealing with at 90 years old—at least, that's what it feels like at this point. For years, I have been saying the same thing over and over again. Misophonia is a real disorder that is not something to make fun of, and yet, the media hasn't gotten this message. I will say that things have gotten better, but as recently as last week I was responding to a tweet by a semi-famous podcast host who asked her followers, "is misophonia real?". I'm not entirely sure why this woman felt the need to question the validity of a condition she clearly knows nothing about, but I digress.

I'm tired of this kind of behavior. Could you imagine if these same people asked, "is autism real?" or "is depression real?". I can't because they would be rightfully shut down. Below is the Twitter poll. I will not share the username because I do not want to blame and shame one person specifically, but the action instead.

Do you believe misophonia is a real problem or a made-up problem?	
Real ⊘	38.5%
Made up	9.5%
It depends	8%
What's that?	44%

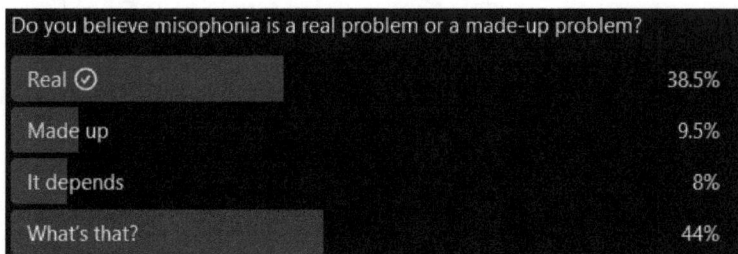

Now, I can't fault these people for not knowing whether or not misophonia exists since it's a newer disorder and it is not yet in the DSM-5. Fine. That's completely true. And yet, a quick search of PubMed would have given them numerous articles that show evidence that the condition is *very real* and incredibly hard for persons with misophonia to live with. At times, I feel like a circus sideshow that's here for the "mildly interesting" crowds who like to poke at weird conditions. Oh, you experience excruciating pain and fight-flight-freeze from chewing, whistling, snoring? How hilarious!

I'm not sure what these social media personas hope to gain by asking if misophonia is real? Engagement on a tweet at the sake of mocking the pain of people they are too lazy to even do a Google search to understand? This reminds me of the time that Kathie Lee and Hoda mocked misophonia and called it "misophoney" while making trigger sounds and laughing.

People with misophonia are experiencing a fight-flight-freeze reaction which then manifests as pain, anger, depression, and impacts quality of life. Can you imagine when your parents, husband, and even kids are causing you distress and pain? Imagine not being able to attend family dinners? Movie theatres? Feeling intense pain in classrooms and having to drop out of school? These are all common things persons with misophonia report.

Misophonia Worksheet

COMMUNICATION EXERCISE

Was there a time in the past where you could have explained misophonia and did not? Why?

_____

_____

_____

_____

_____

_____

_____

_____

_____

We're not your punchline. Please learn more about our disorder and come to this from an educational perspective. This is not a social cause; this is a medical issue. We are *real people* and we come from many walks of life. Before you tweet, please consider the audience. What are you going to gain from this tweet? Who will you hurt?

I will admit that whenever I hear a media personality mock a person with misophonia, or the disorder as a whole, I feel an emotional response. To me, this is a directly offensive remark because I know how awful misophonia feels for those that have the disorder, myself included.

Just a quick Google search away, the 2015 segment "Munch munch: Do certain everyday sounds drive you nuts?" leaves tears in my eyes. Despite a petition after the fact by people with misophonia, the video remains live. This video, which is crass in nature, has always lingered like a shadow.

Misophonia is a neurological disorder that causes a fight/flight/freeze reaction when faced with otherwise normal audial and visual stimuli. In short, this means things such as whistling, tapping, chewing, leg shaking, and coughing can cause a severe emotional reaction.

Perhaps I should toughen up. I should get over it. This happened on August 20, 2015, so it should no longer be relevant. To me, it is just as relevant as the day it was filmed. 3,210 voices signed a petition saying this was not okay. Mere drops in the water. Our voices were silenced because we are not a majority. As this is a rare disorder, we haven't had the chance to speak for ourselves. We have been mocked, berated, and chastised by the media as "those people that feel rage when they hear chewing." We are much more than that. According to this video, we are not. We are gossip worthy, entertainment, a spectacle. So long as videos like this are allowed to stand higher than our voices, it remains relevant.

In a world where the media is allowed to be a spectacle, where the President of the United States can mock a disabled reporter, I am worried I am grasping at straws by speaking of this injustice. I worry daily that our message will not be heard. Misophonia has caused pain to people and families. These stories have become the backdrop for clickbait and entertainment, and on the better days, we remain completely ignored by the press. Even news about research is met with follow-up stories that care little about breakthroughs, science, and the validation of a disorder that many believed to be "made up." No, it seems to me what they care about is the strange affliction of "chewing rage."

Kathie Lee and Hoda have a voice. They have a television show that reaches audiences across North America. I believe they have lent their voice to stigmatization, to the opposition of kindness, compassion, and health awareness. For the sake of entertainment, they have mocked misophonia.

I worry not because these words have been said. I worry because in the world we live in, bigger is often thought of as better. Unfortunately, for those of us struggling in the corners of medicine, with disorders that are unknown, our platforms are smaller. Often, we may feel as though we are shouting in the wind, looking for a sign that we are more than a story. We are people who are struggling with a life-altering disorder. We are struggling every day with isolation, anger, fear, and confusion. We are struggling because our minds do not match our environments. We are struggling because we are unable to adapt to the world around us.

It feels like the media has turned its back on us. There are also under-researched stories about misophonia that link back to individuals I believe wish to profit off the pain of people with misophonia. Giving a voice to the wrong sources can have devastating impacts on disorders that are unknown. Dr. Jennifer Jo Brout, an advocate for misophonia and founder of the IMRN (International Misophonia Research

Network), spoke of this in an article featured by the Observer.

"I've seen a lot of BS treatments for many conditions, but the difference here is that these fraudsters monopolized this disorder. They got to the internet first, before academia and before any doctors, and positioned themselves as experts. When you Google misophonia, you get them. When you read mainstream articles about misophonia, you see their treatments and groups referenced in the articles. Instead of informed doctors or researchers, you find people promising "cures" to desperate sufferers. I know people who have been have bilked out of over $10,000 (and more), never mind the emotional cost incurred."

Advocates for all disorders should be horrified by this behavior. There was once a time when depression, anxiety, and many other disorders were unheard of. There was once a time when it was "OK" to say cruel words on television about persons who are disenfranchised. If we ignore ignorance and cruelty, I am afraid we are riding a slippery slope. Time is a fickle thing. Every decision we make can lead us right back to past moments we thought were left behind us. If we are not careful, we will live in a time where this is okay.

I have tears when I think about this video because I am fighting every day for the opportunity to live my life normally. I am fighting to function in a world that constantly berates me with stimuli. I am fighting against a society that is unequipped to understand my disorder. I face doctors who do not understand. All of us with this disorder have faced parents, teachers, and medical professionals, and have been left with more questions than answers.

Misophonia Worksheet

MONITORING YOUR HEART RATE

Monitor your heart rate once per day for one week while you are in a neutral calm state.

1.

2.

3.

4.

5.

6.

7.

Monitor your heart rate once per day for one week while you are in an anxious state, but you are still able to stay in the room.

1.

2.

3.

4.

5.

6.

7.

Monitor your heart rate while you are triggered and experiencing distress. Since this is hopefully less common and variable, simply do so when it happens and not at a set interval.

_____

_____

_____

Compare the results to assess your baseline state, anxious state, and maximum tolerance level.

Baseline:

Anxious:

Maximum Tolerance:

MISOPHONIA ON TV

As I turned on "Dear White People: Volume 2," the last thing I expected to hear was the word "misophonia." I had to go back and listen again, certain my overly sensitive hearing had failed me. Unfortunately, it had not. The conversation was between Sam and her best friend Joelle as they walked through their satirized Ivy League campus. The show makes a point of zooming in on flip-flops, a noise frustratingly unbearable for those of us who live with misophonia in real life.

"When does the constant drone of flip-flops become background noise?" Joelle asks. A strange question for anybody who has misophonia, since we know it never will. Joelle continues and exclaims, "My misophonia is triggered as fuck."

As Joelle complains, there is no obvious pain on her face. Joelle does not seem to freeze, a particularly telling sign of the fight/flight/freeze reaction. In fact, Joelle seems relatively fine.

"Oh, misophonia? She does braids out of Waller, right?" Sam quips.

"Oh, look at you, making jokes," Joelle says, barely offended, she continues, "It's a hearing condition, and also a great name for an Outkast album." Just like that, misophonia was made into a quick, witty, original joke.

Those who haven't heard of misophonia might be intrigued, thinking what a strange fact that people are bothered by flip-flops? Joelle's reaction, and the subsequent banter between her and Sam make for a funny exchange. However, I don't find misophonia. Misophonia is rarely that easy to tolerate. It is not an annoyance at flip-flops, chewing, or any other sound.

Misophonia involves a great level of emotional fatigue and pain. As I continued to watch the episode, my awareness now heightened, I wondered if this plot point would come up again throughout the episode. I wasn't surprised that it hadn't. Our character Joelle, supposedly having misophonia, is now living with Sam in a dorm room. I am sure there are persons with misophonia that have roommates, but I personally cannot imagine living in such a small space with a potential trigger. Sam's phone notifications go off constantly, and she types on her computer all night. Joelle says nothing and sleeps blissfully throughout the ordeal. Joelle later eats chips (a major trigger for many with misophonia) with Sam, also chomping down on the crispy snack. Joelle goes so far as to buy Sam a pair of flip flops for the shower, the same item used as a plot device for our one-off joke on misophonia. There is almost no representation of misophonia in popular culture. I'd argue it has never once been accurately portrayed.

The problem with the "Dear White People" misophonia reference is that their character likely does not have misophonia. Joelle's and Sam's conversation about misophonia is telling. There is a very real conversation that people with misophonia have with their friends when bringing up the condition for the first time. It is rarely a calm conversation—it is a hard talk, often filled with heightened emotions and pain. Many are met with disbelief—far worse than a joke. Misophonia is not about the annoyance of flip-flops, it is much more. The misery of our condition, including the isolation, is hard to show on television. However, misophonia is more than a quick joke. We are real people who are struggling. While it's great we are starting to see more awareness, without context, this does little more than cause people to question if it's even a real thing. I think back to Kathie Lee and Hoda making fun of misophonia on live television, "it sounds like 'misophoney,'" they said as they laughed.

Coming so soon after the "Criminal Minds" episode, which incorrectly classified misophonia as a psychological disorder, I find this deeply concerning. Awareness for misophonia without context might very well prove to be damaging. While exposure to the name "misophonia" could help people get diagnosed, I wonder at what cost?

Out of all the representations of misophonia, which are few and far between, "Dear White People" didn't do too badly. The problem was a lack of context. Misophonia is not necessarily a "hearing disorder," but the general public won't necessarily notice a large difference between a "hearing disorder" and a neurological disorder involving auditory processing. This is understandable. The representation falls flat when the character exclaims brazenly that her misophonia is "triggered as fuck," the same way a person who is frustrated their car keys weren't left in the right place might say their "OCD is acting up." Neither have the condition they are mirroring. While "Dear White People" trivializes misophonia, I am thankful they did not focus on the rage, specifically "chewing rage," and did make an earnest attempt to mention the condition on TV.

However, I am not happy that popular culture is starting to use a very real condition as the brunt of a joke. Those with misophonia need to keep talking about it from a real perspective. When we speak of the disorder, we must ensure we are encouraging an accurate representation. Unfortunately, in today's society it's very easy to create a meme about how "frustrated" we are, and we end up being minimized to generalized sound bites.

Misophonia Worksheet

NEGOTIATING BOUNDARIES

Unfortunately, there are often triggers that cannot be avoided by the person with misophonia. An example of this is somebody who clears their throat or snores (barring sleep apnea which should get checked out). Some sounds are necessary. More than that, some sounds (and visuals) are part of activities that are important to our partners. This chart is meant to help couples negotiate their "Never", "Sometimes", and "Adapting" triggers. Adapting sounds are ones that are necessary or unavoidable. The adapting portion comes in to help the couple negotiate ways for the misophonia sufferer to live in this environment where triggers are present. The following example is my own chart based on my own triggers, but each couple will have a chart tailored to their situations. These categories can change over time! For example, restaurants used to be in my "Never" category. This list should not be treated like scripture but rather used for couples to identify their needs and boundaries.

Never	Sometimes	Adapting

AWARENESS

Since misophonia is only a newly recognized condition, it is important that the doctors who study it, and the people who suffer from it, are advocating for awareness. Some believe that awareness will lead to negative individuals acting inappropriately against sufferers, but with proper advocacy, this should be alleviated.

Awareness is important for all disorders and conditions. This is evident in the growing support for mental illness and the need for open dialogue and understanding. Of course, it is impossible for the entire world to change in order to help those who have misophonia, but through awareness we will create further incentives for research and for plans that can genuinely help those with misophonia.

In my own experience, misophonia has been much easier to manage now that I can tell my family and friends what is wrong. Like a good diet, healthy and understanding friends and family can lead to an overall improvement in quality of life. It's important that the people you interact with know that there is currently no cure. Therapy might help, but it will not eliminate symptoms.

Once upon a time, many of the disorders we are now aware of and actively working to alleviate today were considered abnormal and strange. Misophonia may currently be considered abnormal or strange, but as awareness grows, this may become a stigma of the past. There may be an initial period of downfall. The more awareness grows, the more it may be considered odd and a piece of gossip. All things must go through this phase. In order to have gains we must be prepared for the potential losses.

Awareness isn't some magical concept that can be achieved simply by wanting it to happen. If we want misophonia to be a widely understood and accepted condition, we must be willing to talk about it. Like all illnesses that have been stigmatized, it starts with a conversation.

It can be difficult to talk about misophonia. There's a lot of pressure when you know that the person on the receiving end probably won't understand what you're going through. That doesn't mean you shouldn't try. Everyone can help raise awareness for misophonia. It starts with your family and friends, your community, your school or workplace. At first, it may be seen as a strange word, a strange disorder, or an annoyance. Over time, it will grow to be something familiar.

Information and exposure are the only way that a person's mind can be changed. Of course, there will always be the naysayers, the doubters, and the people who refuse to respect your illness, but these people exist in all lifestyles, for all reasons. There was once a time when it was okay to label a disabled person as retarded. Now, that's so unspeakable that I considered using asterisks for some of the letters. There was also a time when people with depression and anxiety were told to suck it up, and there was a time just a few decades ago when these people may have spent their lives in an asylum. The world is changing, but it isn't changing through suffering in silence.

It is my belief that access to information is an important way to spread word about this illness. Posts that can be shared, posts featuring information and graphic images, can help those who suffer from misophonia to share information with their friends and families. For me, what's most important is that people know that this is more than a condition and a label; misophonia is a life-altering disorder that can seriously impede a person's quality of life. This book was written for the purpose of awareness. It is through information that we will change how the world views this disorder.

In *Beyond The Label*, stigma is discussed in detail. Stigma is more than just how a person feels about a disorder, as it has a great impact on the life of the sufferer. While misophonia is not the same as mental illness, there is little else to compare it to, and since the reactions appear mental (to an onlooker), it can be put under the same umbrella as many mental illnesses. Below is the definition of stigma in a book designated to raising awareness and cutting away the label for mental illness and addiction.

Stigma is not merely a problem of "hurting people's feelings." Stigma interferes with the person's full participation in society, can lead to and/or increase mental health and substance use problems, and can provoke the person to withdraw from relationships and services that could be helpful. Stigma can seriously hamper matters such as holding a job, having a home, accessing services, and participating in social relationships (CAMH).

The fear of being judged and scrutinized can stop people from looking for help. Since misophonia is not a well-known condition, attempting to search for a cure can be very isolating, which may be worsened when sufferers find out there is none. This is why awareness is so important. Awareness can remove stigma, both from the medical community and from the public. Without research, misophonia will remain a relatively unknown condition, and without advocacy, demand will remain low. The more doctors, graduate students, and laypeople have heard of

misophonia, the greater the chance of finding meaningful treatment or helping sufferers to handle the disorder properly.

Here are some ways that you can help raise awareness for misophonia.

SOCIAL MEDIA

You may think that social media's best attributes are sharing game invites with friends and connecting with your long-lost childhood friends. That may be true, but it also offers a plethora of resources for raising awareness. The ability to post, like, and share has allowed many organizations to get their messages across. The more that people hear about misophonia, the greater the chance that doctors and researchers will learn about it.

Social media is an amazingly powerful platform. Anybody, anywhere, at any time, can connect and share a vision and an idea. It is easy to spread awareness and content with people whom you may never have met without social media. Through Twitter, Google +, and Facebook you can reach a wider audience and ensure that the message of misophonia gets out there. I recommend that you follow the Misophonia International/Misophonia Education page on these sites and share our content with your friends and families.

YOUR COMMUNITY

You may be surprised to learn that your own community holds opportunities to raise awareness. You can ask to set up an information booth at functions, whether these are BBQs, advocacy events, or merely community parties. You can raise a lot of awareness by having pamphlets, posters, and other items ready to promote awareness.

FRIENDS AND FAMILY

Your friends and family can constitute a great backdrop for explaining your disorder. Remember that each person you inform will be able to tell another, and then another. Simply explaining misophonia to others can be both cathartic and a way to spread awareness.

YOUR SCHOOL/WORKPLACE

Like the sources mentioned above, you may be surprised about the awareness you can spread just by talking to your workmates/classmates and other professionals. These people may also have great resources that you can take advantage of. This provides a wonderful opportunity for networking. Moreover, you never know what somebody will be working on down the road, and how you can be mutually beneficial to one another.

WRITE YOUR ARTICLE

Writing articles about misophonia can be a very therapeutic process. By writing an article about misophonia, you are able to process your stressors and tell your story. Whether you write this article to publish or simply for your own journal, this process is one of exploration of your disorder. If you like, this article can even be published on your own blog or submitted to Misophonia International. This is entirely optional, but always available to members of the misophonia community to share our stories and learn from one another.

THINGS YOU COULD INCLUDE IN YOUR ARTICLE.

- How misophonia impacts you.
- How you cope with misophonia.
- What people without misophonia should know.
- What would you tell somebody who just learned about misophonia?
- Tell a particular story about misophonia (for example, living with misophonia when sick; living with misophonia at college).

The point of the article is to reflect on your point of view regarding misophonia while refocusing from a more neutral standpoint. Consider the audience as you write, rather than yourself.

EXAMPLE ARTICLE

This example article was one that I personally used for coping with misophonia half a decade ago.

THE LIFE OF A YOUNG ADULT WITH MISOPHONIA

Like a ghost, the memory of finger-tapping has become my own personal poltergeist. I feel jolted just as one would if the doors were slamming—if the lights were erratically going on and off.

I lie in bed and I replay each finger tap. I do not want to think about it—but like bullets from a gun I replay every second. Bump. Bump. The ferocity echoes through my brain—the noise, god the noise—it is just as loud as it was in person.

At twenty-four years old, I should be living every moment of my life to the fullest. I should be partying, making mistakes, and spending long wistful nights walking barefoot in the park. I should be kissing strangers in alleyways, because I am young and mistakes are part of what makes life worth living. I should be drinking a little too much and stumbling home just before the sun rises. I have a desire to do these things. I want to be young and careless. I want to go out for the night without prior planning, and I want to live my life to the fullest. Instead, I am trapped. I am locked into a world that is dictated by a disorder that suffocates my lust for life. Every decision is marred by its touch. I have gone to clubs, and I have had some fun, but I am increasingly losing my ability to be young and carefree. Instead, I am young and restless.

I have misophonia. While the internet is busy classifying us as a strange, weird, or violent disorder, the truth is a little more depressing. It is true that many of us are upset by chewing—but this disorder goes much further than frustration when our family members crunch down on potato chips. Many of us often struggle from sensory problems similar to that of Sensory Processing Disorder. This disorder is more than an aversion to sounds—it is an all-encompassing prison.

The strangest part is that when there are no sounds, I am normal. It is as though the disorder has evaporated. I am still myself. I will be going about my life like everybody else. I walk like a person that has never been troubled. Everything is fine. Until it is not.

Imagine for a second that you are trapped in a cave with a dripping faucet. This faucet would continue and eventually become torture. For those of us with misophonia, we are immediately trapped in the cave. Because of our amygdala, we do not get used to sounds. Instead, we are bombarded by a fight-flight-freeze response. We are constantly sick, anxious, and living in a world where our bodies are sensorily taxed. Much deeper than simple anger, we are often isolated from our lives. There is no cure for misophonia, and increased exposure can make the disorder worse. Because of this, and the cycle of pain and anxiety, we are more likely to avoid unnecessary social events. Further than that, if I were to "push myself", I am likely to end up with a severe migraine.

The normal life of a twenty-four-year-old is something I am not going to have. It has taken some time to adjust to the idea that, unless the research of the Misophonia and Emotion Regulation Program of Duke is successful, I may be living with this severe condition for much of my adult life. Truth be told, I am terrified. The life of a young adult with misophonia is a confusing one. I have not been out, or partied, in over a year. Since social groups are often how we define our youth—I have had to find interests that are solitary. I have not been on a date in a year either. As the disorder worsens, my interests have been chipped away one by one—the memory of events, and the risk of them repeating, has been the deciding factor in many of my activities.

If I were to go on a date, it would have to be something small and solitary. Movie theatres, due to the popcorn, leg-shaking, and loud noises, are simply impossible. Restaurants also have chewing, and I generally avoid any situation where people are sitting down. Sitting in a car can be hard if the person rests their arm on the windowsill or taps their fingers on the car wheel. I cannot control my fight-flight-freeze reaction, and it is hard to explain to others why it is happening when there are little resources and awareness to point them to—I am exasperated as I try to explain that it is not them I am mad at, but the sound itself is causing my brain to go into overdrive and short circuit. Sadly, it has become easier to not explain at all. To simply stay home and control what is going to happen.

A day for me usually begins with the night. During normal daytime hours there are honking horns, lawnmowers, buzzing motors, screaming children, and persons that inevitably may show up at the door. Instead, I have opted for a life that takes place during the hours of 8PM and 10AM. There are still noises, even in this sheltered life. Even in a world that is considered rural compared to cities. No days are without triggers, and as these triggers mount, I become sick. After triggers, my muscles tense so tight that I have back pain, I become nauseated and dizzy. If I do not remove myself from the situation, these symptoms become worse. The longest migraine from misophonia that I have had was 7 days long. When dealing with reactions this strong, avoidance becomes the main tool in your arsenal.

The world of misophonia and over-responsivity means that some clothes are too tight, lights are far too bright, and we are more likely to get migraines. Scent allergies are common, and perfume can quickly make us sick. Visuals can cause the fight-flight-freeze response too. Effectively, we are being threatened by everyday occurrences at a level that can be hard to explain—we are also attacked by media that is convinced we are overreacting or are a "think-piece". After all, it is strange and unruly to think that the regular world could be causing people so much distress. Unfortunately, I am here to tell you that this condition is very real.

The life of a young adult with misophonia is the life of a girl who was making As and Bs in university her first term—then, as triggers grew, attendance dropped. Eventually, to continue at all, I had to switch to online school. I became so suffocated by the triggers that I could not hear what was going on in the classroom. To even survive the class, I would have to distract myself—and nothing was enough to distract from pen clicking, from legs shaking, and other students that were simply trying to learn. For me, I was trying to survive. Like many other young adult experiences, the college life was another that I had to step back from. While I am still finishing my degree online, it is taking much longer. The social connection and wonderful memories that accompanied my first year have been replaced by my bedroom and textbooks. While I love learning, there is a loss that has taken place.

Misophonia is not chewing rage, sound rage, or "murderous rage". Misophonia is loneliness. It is the loss of social relationships and the decaying of what we could have been, or what we used to be. Misophonia is a daily fight and struggle. We must remain hopeful despite every life change, despite the sickness, and despite being trapped in fight-flight-freeze much of our days. Misophonia is resilience, because if we can survive this and still accomplish some of our goals, we have fought the toughest battle of all—the battle against our own brains.

Misophonia Worksheet

TURNING MISOPHONIA INTO FICTION

Turning misophonia into fiction has been very therapeutic in my own life. In fact, I wrote an entire novel which showcases a character with misophonia. I am not saying that you need to write a novel, nor do you even need to write a cohesive story. The idea is that you take your misophonia and instead of writing from your own perspective, you create a character through which you can process these emotions. You might be surprised where your imagination takes you in your fictitious scenario. The idea is to write without planning and allow your imagination to take you places you were not expecting.

Your Fiction

_____

_____

_____

_____

_____

_____

_____

_____

_____

_____

_____

_____

_____

_____

_____

_____

_____

_____

CONCLUSION

The goal this book set out to achieve was to help teens and adults with misophonia understand their condition better and to find reasonable ways to cope with misophonia. Hopefully, you were able to find something in this book that helped alleviate the severity of your misophonia. If not, I want to leave you on a note of hope that research is continuing and misophonia literature is an ever-growing field. I have seen great strides made in the past decade, and I believe this will only continue to pick up speed and grow.

For those who are interested in participating in misophonia research studies, I encourage you to visit the International Misophonia Foundation website at www.misophoniafoundation.com to view our on-going studies. It is our hope that as a community we can help add our own perspective to research and help academics understand the complexities of our condition through misophonia-sufferer-led studies that are designed with our interests in mind.

REFERENCES

Ayres, A. J. (1968). Sensory integrative processes and neuropsychological learning disability. *Learning Disorders,* 3.

Ayres, A. J. (1972). *Sensory integration and learning disorders.* Los Angeles: Western Psychological Services.

Ayres, A. J. (1979). *Sensory integration and the child.* Los Angeles: Western Psychological Services.

The Bowen Center for the Study of the Family. (n.d.). https://www.thebowencenter.org/

Brout, J.J., Edelstein, M., Erfanian, M., Mannino, M., Miller, L.J., Rouw, R., Kumar, S., & Rosenthal, M.Z. (2018). Investigating misophonia: A review of the empirical literature, clinical implications, and a research agenda. *Frontiers in Neuroscience*, 12(36).

Brout, J.J. (2021). A clinician's guide to understanding and managing misophonia from a self-regulation perspective: Regulate, reason, reassure. *The International Misophonia Research Network.*

Dunn, W. (2014). Sensory profile 2. Bloomington, MN, USA: Psych Corporation.

Jager, I.J., Vulink, N.C.C., Bergfeld, I.O., van Loon, A.J.J.M., & Denys, D.A.J.P. (2021). Cognitive behavioral therapy for misophonia: A randomized clinical trial. *Depression and Anxiety,* 38(7).

Jastreboff, M. M., & Jastreboff, P. J. (2001). Components of decreased sound tolerance: Hyperacusis, misophonia, phonophobia. *ITHS Newsletter.*

Kumar, S., Tansley-Hancock, O., Sedley, W., Winston, J.S., Callaghan, M.F., Allen, M., Cope, T.E., Gander, P.E.,

Bamiou, D.E., & Griffiths, T.D. (2017). The brain basis for misophonia. *Current Biology, 27*(4).

Kumar, S., Dheerendra, P., Erfanian, M., Benzaquén, E., Sedley, W., Gander, P.E., Lad, M., Bamiou, D.E., & Griffiths, T.D. (2021). The motor basis for misophonia. *Journal of Neuroscience, 41*(26).

LeBouef, T., Yaker, Z., & Whited, L. (2023). Physiology, autonomic nervous system. *StatPearls Publishing.* https://www.ncbi.nlm.nih.gov/books/NBK538516/

Miller, L.J., Nielsen, D.M., Schoen, S.A., & Brett-Green, B.A. (2009). Perspectives on sensory processing disorder: A call for translational research. *Frontiers in Integrative Neuroscience, 3*(22).

Miller, L.J., Marco, E.J., Chu, R.C., & Camarata, S. (2021). Editorial: sensory processing across the lifespan: A 25-year initiative to understand neurophysiology, behaviors, and treatment effectiveness for sensory processing. *Frontiers in Integrative Neuroscience,* 15.

Moncrieff, J. (2018). Against the stream: Antidepressants are not antidepressants—An alternative approach to drug action and implications for the use of antidepressants. *BJPsych Bulletin, 42*(1).

Nesbit, S. (n.d). The sensory diet for adults and teens. *Misophonia International.*

Piccardi, E. S., & Gliga, T. (2022). Understanding sensory regulation in typical and atypical development: The case of sensory seeking. *Developmental Review,* 65.

Porcaro, C.K., Alavi, E., Gollery, T., & Danesh, A.A. (2019). Misophonia: Awareness and responsiveness among academics. *Journal of Postsecondary Education and Disability,* 32(2).

Rinaldi, L.J., Simner, J., Koursarou, S., & Ward, J. (2023). Autistic traits, emotion regulation, and sensory sensitivities in children and adults with misophonia. *Journal of Autism and Developmental Disorders,* 53(3).

Rosenthal, M.Z., Anand, D., Cassiello-Robbins, C., Williams, Z.J., Guetta, R.E., Trumbull, J., & Kelley, L.D. (2021). Development and initial validation of the duke misophonia questionnaire. *Frontiers in Psychology,* 12.

Rosenthal, M.Z., McMahon, K., Greenleaf, A.S., Cassiello-Robbins, C., Guetta, R., Trumbull, J., Anand, D., Frazer-Abel, E.S., & Kelley, L. (2022). Phenotyping misophonia: Psychiatric disorders and medical health correlates. *Frontiers in Psychology,* 13.

Schröder, A., Vulink, N., & Denys, D. (2013). Misophonia: Diagnostic criteria for a new psychiatric disorder. *PLOS ONE,* 8(1).

Schröder, A., van Wingen, G., Eijsker, N., San Giorgi, R., Vulink, N.C., Turbyne, C., & Denys, D. (2019). Misophonia is associated with altered brain activity in the auditory cortex and salience network. *Scientific Reports,* 9(1).

Shanker, S., & Barker, T. (2016). *Self-Reg: How to help your child (and you) break the stress cycle and successfully engage with life.* Canada: Penguin Random House.

Ungvarsky, J. (2022). Bowenian family therapy. *Salem Press Encyclopedia.*

Waxenbaum, J.A., Reddy, V., & Varacallo, M. (2023). Anatomy, autonomic nervous system. *StatPearls Publishing.* https://www.ncbi.nlm.nih.gov/books/NBK539845/

Ahn, R., Miller, L. J., Milberger, S., &McIntosh, D. N. (2004). Prevalence of parents' perceptions of sensory processing disorders among kindergarten children. American Journal of Occupational Therapy, 58 (3), 287-302.

Alvarado, J.C, Vaughan, J.W, Stanford, T.R., and Stein, B.E. (2007). Multisensory Versus Unisensory Integration: Contrasting Modes in the Superior Colliculus. Journal of Neurophysiology 97, 3193–3205.

Ben-Sasson, A., Carter, A.S., & Briggs Gowan, M.J. (2009). Sensory over- responsivity in elementary school: prevalence and social-emotional correlates. Journal of Abnormal Child Psychology, 37, 705-716.

Ben-Sasson, A., Carter, A.S., & Briggs-Gowan, M.J. (2010). The development of sensory over-responsivity from infancy to elementary school. Journal of Abnormal Child Psychology, 38 (8), 1193-1202.

Carter, A.S., Ben-Sasson, A., & Briggs-Gowan, M.J. (2011). Sensory over- responsivity, psychopathology, and family impairment in school-aged children. Journal of the American Academy of Child & Adolescent Psychiatry, 50 (12), 1210-1219.

Davies, P.L., Chang, W-P., & Gavin, W.J. (2009). Maturation of Sensory Gating Performance in Children with and without Sensory Processing Disorders. International Journal of Psychophysiology, 72, 187-197.

Davies P.L., Chang, W.P., & Gavin, W.J. (2010). Middle and late latency ERP components discriminate between adults, typical children, and children with sensory processing disorders. Frontiers in Integrative Neuroscience, 4, 16.

Davies, P.L. & Gavin, W.J. (2007). Validating the diagnosis of Sensory Processing Disorders using EEG technology. American Journal of Occupational Therapy, 61 (2), 176-189.

Edelstein, M., Brang, D., Rouw, R., Ramachandran, V.S. (2013). Misophonia: physiological investigations and case descriptions. Frontiers in Human Neuroscience 2013;7(296), 1-11, doi: 10.3389/fnhum.2013.00296.

Gavin, W. J., Dotseth, A., Roush, K. K., Smith, C. A., Spain, H. D., & Davies, P. L. (2011). Electroencephalography in children with and without sensory processing disorders during auditory perception. American Journal of Occupational Therapy, 65, 370–377.

Goldsmith, H.H., Van Hulle, C.A., Arneson, C.L., Schreiber, J.E., & Gernsbacher, M.A. (2006). A population-based twin study of parentally reported tactile and auditory defensiveness in young children. Journal of Abnormal Child Psychology, 34 (3), 393-407.

Jastreboff, M.M., Jastreboff, P.J. (2001) Hyperacusis. Audiology Online. www.audiologyonline.com/articles/hyperacusis-1223.

Jastreboff, P.J., Jastreboff, M.M. (2006) Tinnitus retraining therapy: a different view on tinnitus. International Journal of Pediatric Otorhinolaryngology, 68 (1), 23–29.

Keuler, M.M., Schmidt, N.L., Van Hulle, C.A., Lemery-Chalfant, K., & Goldsmith, H.H. (2011). Sensory overresponsivity: prenatal risk factors and temperamental contributions. Journal of Development & Behavioral Pediatrics, 32 (7), 533-541.

Kisley, M.A., Noecker, L., Guinther, P.M. (2004).
Comparison of sensory gating to mismatch negativity
and self-reported perceptual phenomena in healthy
adults. International Journal of Psychophysiology, 41,
604–612. doi: 10.1111/j.1469-8986.2004.00191.x.

Lane, S.J., Reynolds, S., & Thacker, L. (2010). Sensory over-
responsivity and ADHD: differentiating using
electrodermal responses, cortisol, and anxiety.
Frontiers in Integrative Neuroscience, 4 (8), 1-14.
doi:10.3389/ fnint.2010.00008.

McIntosh, D.N., Miller, L.J., Shyu, V., Hagerman. (1999).
Sensory-modulation disruption, electrodermal
responses, and functional behaviors. Developmental
Medicine & Child Neurology, 41, 608-615.

Owen, J.P., Marco E.J., Desai S., Fourie E., Harris J., Hill
S.S., Arnett A.B., Mukherjee P., (2103) Abnormal
white matter microstructure in children with sensory
processing disorders. NeuroImage: Clinical, 2, 844–
853.

Rosenthal, M.Z., Ahn, R. & Geiger, P.J. (2011). Reactivity to
Sensations in Borderline Personality Disorder: A
Preliminary Study. Journal of Personality Disorders,
(25), 5, 715-721.

Schaaf, R.C., Miller, L.J., Seawell, D., & O'Keefe, S. (2003).
Children with disturbances in sensory processing: A
pilot study examining the role of the parasympathetic
nervous system. American Journal of Occupational
Therapy, 57.

Schneider, M.L., Moore, C.F., Larson, J.A., Barr, C.S.,
DeJesus, O.T., & Roberts, A.D. (2009). Timing of
moderate level of prenatal alcohol exposure
influences gene expression of sensory processing

behavior in rhesus monkeys. Frontiers in Integrative Neuroscience, 3, 30.

Schröder, A., Vulink, N., Denys, D. (2013) Misophonia: diagnostic criteria for a new psychiatric disorder. PLoS One, 8 (1). doi: 10.1371/journal.pone. 0054706.

Tavassoli, T., Miller, L.J., Schoen, S.A.Nielsen, D.M. &Baron-Cohen S. (2014). Sensory over-responsivity in adults with autism spectrum conditions. Autism, 18 (4), 28-32.

Van Hulle, C.A., Schmidt, N.L., & Goldsmith, H.H. (2012). Is sensory over- responsivity distinguishable from childhood behavior problems? A phenotypic and genetic analysis. Journal of Child Psychology and Psychiatry, 53 (1), 64-72.

Wu, M.S., Lewin A.B., Murphy, T.K., Storch, E.A. (2014) Misophonia: incidence, phenomenology, and clinical correlates in an undergraduate student sample. Journal of Clinical Psychology. Published online April 17. doi: 10.1002/jclp.22098.

Shaylynn Hayes-Raymond is a Licensed Counselling Therapist Candidate in New Brunswick, Canada and has been an advocate for misophonia and mental illness since 2015.

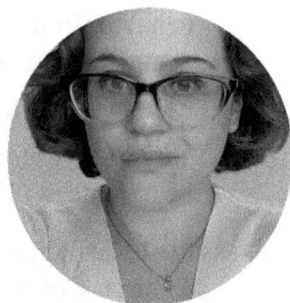

Shaylynn is passionate about providing accessible mental healthcare through telehealth therapy and is particularly interested in working with clients with misophonia, OCD, PTSD, depression, career counselling, and general life struggles. Shaylynn is the Director of The International Misophonia Foundation and is continuing her advocacy and research through the foundation. Shaylynn provides counselling services in Canada and coaching services worldwide. You can find more information about these services on her personal website at www.shaylynnraymond.com.

www.ingramcontent.com/pod-product-compliance
Lightning Source LLC
Chambersburg PA
CBHW062132020426
42335CB00013B/1194